THE PROSTATE CANCER ESSENTIALS FOR SURVIVAL SERIES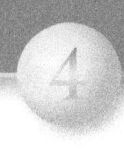

INTERPRETING YOUR PSA RESULTS

AND RELATED PROSTATE CANCER LAB TESTS

MICHAEL J. DATTOLI, MD

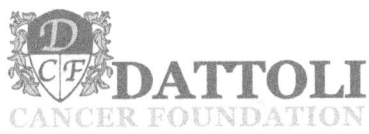

SARASOTA, FLORIDA

Prostate Cancer Essentials for Survival: Interpreting Your PSA Results and Related Prostate Cancer Lab Tests

Copyright © 2020–2026 by Michael J. Dattoli, M.D.

All rights reserved. No part of this work may be reproduced or transmitted in any form or by any means, electronic or mechanical, including photocopying or recording, or by any information storage or retrieval system, except as may be expressly permitted by the 1976 Copyright Act or in writing by the publisher.

ISBN-10: 1-9877266-8-5
ISBN-13: 978-1-9877-2668-8

Published by the Dattoli Cancer Foundation, Sarasota, FL
Book design and composition by Daniel van Loon, Batavia, IL
Book edits and revisions by Design Corps, Colorado Springs, CO

MEDICAL DISCLAIMER

This booklet is intended as a supplement but not as a substitute for the medical advice of a physician. It is imperative that you consult a qualified healthcare professional with regard to all matters relating to your health and particular situation. Neither the publisher nor the authors bear responsibility for any consequences due to the reader's decision to use any particular treatment, medication, dietary supplement or other healthcare practices discussed in this book.

DEDICATION

This booklet is dedicated to all those whose lives have been touched by prostate cancer, and to the patients and their families whom we are privileged to serve and educate as cancer care providers.

ACKNOWLEDGMENTS

We are deeply grateful to a number of people who have contributed to this booklet in a number of ways. Our thanks to Greg Lawrence, for his editorial efforts and to Ginya Carnahan, Chris Wells, and Jone Fay for their ongoing assistance.

With this booklet, we are also indebted to Jennifer Undella, MLT, ASCP for her survey on current blood assays and lab testing.

We deeply appreciate all of those wonderful patients and family members who have contacted the Dattoli Cancer Foundation for counseling and guidance and in turn have given us their support and encouragement. It is your spirit and commitment in confronting this disease that inspires us all.

CONTENTS

INTRODUCTION—TO SCREEN OR NOT TO SCREEN 9

OVERVIEW—THE PSA AND OTHER BLOOD TESTS 12

- What is the PSA Test? 13
- What is the Digital Rectal Exam (DRE)? 14
- How are PSA Results Reported? 15
- Why is there Controversy about PSA Screening? 18
- What is PSA Velocity? 19
- What are Free and Bound PSA? 20
- What is PSA Density? 21
- What is the PAP Test? 21
- What is the PCA3Plus™ Test? 22
- What is a Prostate Biopsy and How is it Performed? 23
- Dr. Dattoli on Anesthetic Techniques Utilized for Painless Prostate Biopsies 25
- What is the Gleason Score? 26
- What is DNA Ploidy Analysis? 27
- How are Biopsy Results Reported? 27
- What is Transrectal Ultrasound (TRUS)? 28
- What are CT Scans and Fused Imaging Modalities? 29
- What is Magnetic Resonance Imaging (MRI) and How Does It Work? 30
- What are Multiparametric MRI and PI-RADS Analysis? 30
- Dattoli Team Biopsy Results with Color-flow Doppler Ultrasound 34
- What is a Bone Scan? 36
- What are the ProstaVysion and QuadVysion™ Tests? 36

APPENDICES 41

A: References and Abstracts *41*
B: A Survey of Currently Available Blood Tests and Their Uses *45*
C: Deciding What is Best for You *53*
D: Glossary of Medical Terms *55*
E: The Warning Signs of Prostate Cancer *69*

About the Author *70*
Dattoli Cancer Foundation Mission *71*
Order More Booklets in the Series *72*

INTRODUCTION

TO SCREEN OR NOT TO SCREEN

In recent years, the PSA blood test, which is used in screening for prostate cancer, has sparked considerable controversy in the media and in the medical community. The purpose of this booklet is to help men become fully informed and understand the issues when making their personal choice about whether or not to undergo PSA testing and related lab tests that may be indicated. Directly related to the issue of which men should be screened for prostate cancer is the question of which men should be treated for the disease. Age, overall health and risk factors need to be taken into account.

Some prostate cancers are indolent and may not require treatment, while others are life-threatening and should be treated. Determining the appropriate course of action can be a dilemma for both doctors and patients, one that can only be resolved with a comprehensive regime of lab tests, including the PSA blood test.

In the past, it was argued that prostate cancer patients with a life expectancy less than 10 years should not be treated, because they were more likely to die from some other cause. But with life expectancy increasing again in 2020, there are actually only a relatively small percentage of cases of prostate cancer these days that do not call for some form of treatment. Older men should be evaluated on a case by case basis. In 2006, SEER-Medicare data demonstrate a significant survival advantage for patients (ages 65 to 80) treated with radiation or surgery compared to patients who were not treated (Wong YN, et al, "Survival associated with treatment vs observation of localized prostate cancer in elderly men," (JAMA, 2006 Dec 13;296(22):2683-93). Relatively noninvasive treatments, such as the most advanced radiation therapies, brachytherapy and/or Dynamic Adaptive Radiotherapy (DART) are often appropriate for older men, including those over 75, who are otherwise in good health—with less risk of surgical side effects that may reduce quality of life.

Another study has shown that in the early 1990s as a result of PSA screening, the U.S. and U.K. had the same incidence of prostate cancer per capita; but since that time the U.S. has enjoyed more than a 4-fold decline in mortality compared to the

U.K. And this was attributed directly to our treating elderly patients with definitive therapies vs watchful waiting, as is the method of choice in the U.K. (Lancet Oncol. 2008 May;9(5):407-9).

With regard to life expectancy, we often see reports in the media that offer life tables that indicate American males are living an average of 75.8 years, but that's measured from birth. If you're already 70 years of age, you have a 14.7-year life expectancy. This was data reported in 2025 based on data from 2023 *(National Vital Statistics Reports, Vol. 74, No. 6, July 15, 2025)*. In the case of an 80-year-old whose general health is good and who has no other serious health conditions, he stands a good chance of living beyond 10 years and would be wise to consider treatment for prostate cancer. A man's overall health should be considered as well as his age, since an 84 year old may actually be healthier than his 54 year old counterpart who smokes cigarettes, consumes excessive alcohol, etc.

While many doctors continue to use 10 years life expectancy as a strict benchmark, when biopsy pathology and other lab tests identify aggressive, potentially life-threatening tumors, a 5-year cutoff may be indicated, and that would suggest screening is appropriate even for many men over the age of 75, who can be effectively treated with radiation and/or hormonal therapy.

In May of 2012, the controversy about PSA screening was reignited when the U.S. Preventative Services Task Force (USPSTF) issued a recommendation against screening for all men regardless of age and risk factors such as race and family history. That guideline was later revised to recommend against screening for all men 70 years of age and older (USPSTF guidelines updated 2018). The recommendations have been widely criticized in the prostate cancer field by many doctors and medical groups, including the Prostate Cancer Roundtable, an association of a dozen not-for-profit prostate cancer organizations. The controversy traces back to 2009 when two studies were published, one in the U.S. and one in Europe (see abstracts in Appendix A). The American study showed no benefits to screening, but it followed patients for only 7 years, not long enough to show significant results in terms of survival. Moreover, that study was shown to be flawed in a number of ways by many researchers in the field, as the trial populations were poorly controlled.

The European study in 2009 was conducted more rigorously, with twice as many patients and a follow-up of 14 years. It showed that deaths from prostate cancer for patients who were screened with the PSA test were 20% fewer than for patients who were not screened (Schroder FH, et al, N Engl J Med, 2009 Mar 26;360(13):1320-8).

Two more European studies in 2010 and 2011 confirmed those landmark European results in dramatic fashion, demonstrating that prostate cancer mortality actually decreased by as much as 50% with screening (see abstracts in Appendix A). Those results received far less media coverage in the U.S. than the previous flawed study.

A more recent retrospective study by a multi-institutional group of researchers reviewed the results of the previous American and European studies and concluded that PSA screening reduced prostate cancer deaths by 25% to 32% ("The efficacy of prostate specific antigen screening: Impact of key components in the ERSPC and PLCO trials," de Koning HJ, et al, Cancer, 2017 Dec 6).

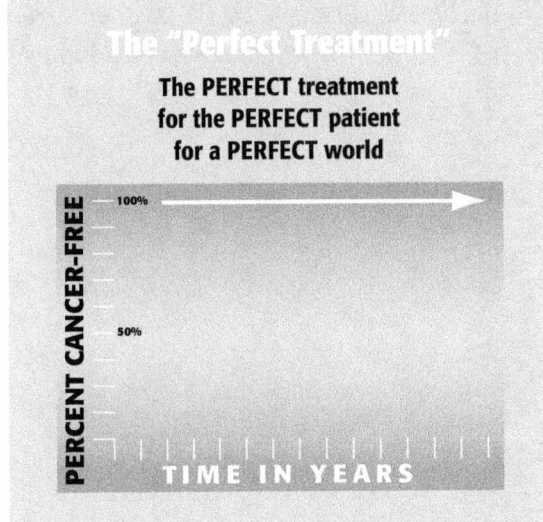

With all of these recent studies in mind, it is essential for you to understand the significance of the PSA test and how to interpret your results—whether you are trying to decide on testing with your doctor, or you are newly diagnosed and struggling to decide which form of treatment, if any, is right for you. The PSA is also used for monitoring a patient's condition after all forms of treatment. Understanding your PSA can help you make informed decisions, as you consult with your doctor, decisions that may very well save your life and lifestyle.

Before being tested, you should know that an abnormal PSA reading may not be the result of cancer. An abnormal result can also be caused by enlargement of the prostate known as benign prostatic hypertrophy (BPH), by infections, by certain drugs and by other causes discussed in greater detail in the pages ahead. Taken by itself, the PSA is not a perfect test, but it can be a red flag indicating that further testing may be appropriate. Interpreted wisely in light of a number of related laboratory tests, the PSA can be a powerful tool for making decisions about when to treat, when not to treat, and which forms of treatment may be most effective in each individual case. It's therefore a good idea to get a reading on your PSA before doing anything else. There are now a number of ways to analyze serum PSA, including total PSA, free PSA, age-adjusted PSA, ethnically adjusted PSA, PSA velocity and PSA density. Each of these tests provides additional insights and has unique characteristics that will be discussed in detail in this booklet

It should be noted that before deciding on any course of treatment, you should fully investigate the likelihood of cure and the risk of side effects that may alter your quality of life. These are the most important considerations in deciding on therapy. Given your age and overall health, you will want to find a balance between treatment effectiveness and side effects—a balance with which you are comfortable, that you can live with both before and after treatment. Knowing what to expect each step of the way is one of the keys to fighting this disease.

—Michael J. Dattoli, M.D., Physician-in-Chief,
Dattoli Cancer Center & Brachytherapy Research Institute

OVERVIEW

THE PSA AND OTHER BLOOD TESTS

What is the PSA Test?

The PSA test was developed during the late 1970s by research scientists at Roswell Park Memorial Hospital in Buffalo, New York. The PSA is a blood test that measures the amount of *prostate specific antigen* (PSA) present in the body. Produced almost exclusively by the prostate gland, PSA is an enzyme, typically present in only minute quantities, secreted into the bloodstream from blood vessels inside the prostate.

PSA secretions originate from cells in the lining of the prostate gland. The function of PSA appears to be liquefying the gelatinous semen and sustaining the viability of the sperm after ejaculation. When prostate cancer is present, additional PSA is usually produced. This extra PSA can be detected and measured in the blood through a simple laboratory test, which can be ordered by any primary-care physician. Test results are usually available in 1-3 days. The test has been widely used since 1990.

Because cancerous cells readily leak PSA into the surrounding body tissue, an elevated PSA is a possible indicator of the presence of prostate cancer. However, other conditions can also cause an elevated PSA. The most common is the enlargement of the prostate gland that occurs with BPH (benign prostatic hyperplasia). Infections and traumas such as a biopsy or even an overly vigorous digital rectal exam can sometimes increase PSA levels. **Ejaculation** (orgasm) can elevate PSA for as long as 48 hours.

Though the PSA test is far from perfect as an indicator of cancer, the American Cancer Society (ACS) suggests that starting at age 50, men should talk to their doctor about the pros and cons of testing so they can decide if testing is the right choice for them. The ACS guidelines also suggest testing may be advisable for men who are considered at higher risk (such as African-American males and those men with a family history of prostate cancer) starting at age 45. For men with even higher risk,

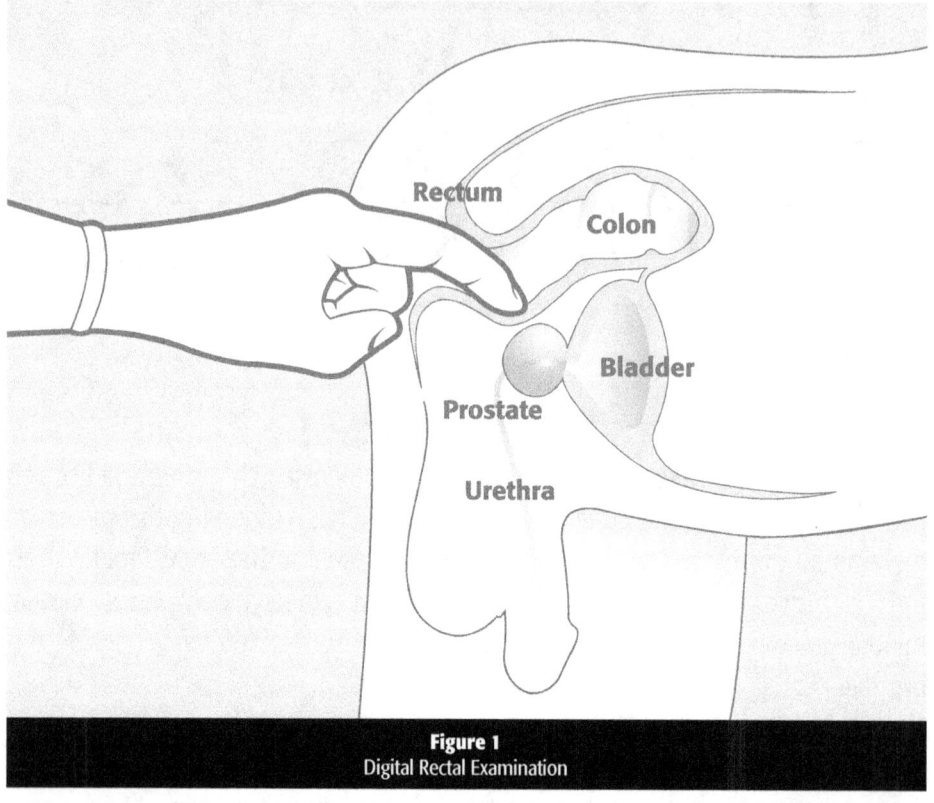

Figure 1
Digital Rectal Examination

such as those with several first-degree relatives who were diagnosed with prostate cancer at an early age, initial testing should be considered by age 40.

As a diagnostic tool, the PSA test has its limitations, and is usually combined with the digital rectal examination (DRE). Some men with apparently normal PSA values turn out to have prostate cancer that may be detected with the DRE or by other lab tests.

What is the Digital Rectal Exam (DRE)?

The digital rectal exam is the simplest way to detect physical abnormalities in the prostate gland that may suggest the presence of cancer. The DRE is also used to estimate the volume of the prostate and the extent of the cancer. The test is part of the physician's *work-up*, which involves a series of laboratory and radiographic tests that are used to determine how advanced the cancer is. The results of these tests will be evaluated to determine the *clinical stage* of the cancer, and they are also used to decide which type of treatment is most appropriate for your particular cancer.

To perform the rectal exam, the doctor feels the gland by placing a lubricated, gloved finger inside the rectum against the prostate. When done properly, the test is not as discomforting as it might sound. Most cancers are located in the back of the prostate, and some of these cancers that have grown at the edge of the gland can be felt as a lump or hard nodule. Depending on the size, shape and location of the lump, it is sometimes possible to determine with a DRE if the cancer has spread beyond the prostate capsule. With the DRE, the doctor is able to evaluate the major portions of the gland's anatomy: the right and left sides or *lobes*; the upper portion or base of the gland; the middle portion of the gland; and lower portion or apex.

Unfortunately, the DRE is often not conclusive. Many prostate cancers do not protrude against the back of the gland; they are not palpable and cannot be detected with the DRE. A tumor at the front of the prostate cannot be felt through the rectum. In addition, the test is subjective and depends on the skill of the doctor, providing at best only an estimate of the extent of disease. Many surgical studies have shown that more than 50% of cancers that appear to be confined to the gland will later be found to have spread outside the prostate gland. Once a tumor is palpable, there are more than a billion cancer cells.

How are PSA Results Reported?

Standard PSA test results are reported in nanograms per milliliter (ng/ml), with a normal range of approximately 0 to 4.0 ng/ml. For the sake of simplicity, the units of measure will not be included in the remainder of this booklet when discussing PSA values. The normal range of PSA values must be adjusted slightly to account for differences in age and race (see box below). As men get older, the normal PSA range slowly increases. This normal range is generally higher for white males than for Asians and African-Americans, who are at greater risk and therefore should make sure that they are monitored closely if the PSA begins to rise or if they have an abnormal DRE.

Regardless of age and race factors, PSA levels greater than 10 are most often an accurate indicator of cancer. As many as 80% of men with this high a PSA reading (and a positive digital rectal exam) have been shown to have prostate cancer (as noted below, at our institution, we are finding an even greater percentage). Approximately 25 percent of those patients with a PSA between 4 and 10 turn out to have cancer. The accuracy of the PSA test is significantly improved when it is combined with the digital rectal exam. The PSA can detect twice as many cancers as the DRE alone; however, the DRE spots some cancers that may be missed by the PSA.

It should be stressed that the PSA test is not conclusive by itself in diagnosing prostate cancer. No treatment decision should ever be made on the basis of the

Table 1
PSA–Typical "Normal" Range by Age & Race

Age	White	Asian	African-American
40-49	0-2.5	0-2.0	0-2.0
50-59	0-3.5	0-3.0	0-4.0
60-69	0-4.5	0-4.0	0-4.5
70-79	0-6.5	0-5.0	0-5.5

PSA value by itself; however, an elevated PSA reading may suggest the need for further laboratory tests. A biopsy of the prostate gland is **always** necessary to confirm the presence of cancer (see below, "What is a Prostate Biopsy?").

Because the PSA test is not completely reliable as far as its predictive value, a patient with a high PSA level may not necessarily have cancer; and a patient with a very low PSA may not be cancer free. In fact, high grade, more aggressive cancers can lose their resemblance to prostate cells altogether and may not even produce PSA. About 20% of men with prostate cancer have PSA scores in the normal range. The PSA provides only a statistical approximation, and there are often exceptions. PSA results are discussed in terms of probabilities–the likelihood of prostate cancer being present, and the likelihood that it may have spread beyond the prostate gland.

At our center, we are often suspicious of any PSA greater than 2.5, especially with men who are 40 to 55 years old; however, we are equally suspicious of a patient who has a normal PSA or even a low PSA, but an abnormal digital rectal examination. For example, if you have a man who has a prostate nodule and his PSA is 1.2, that's worth looking into with further testing. It may become even more concerning if he tells us that his father had prostate cancer or his brother had prostate cancer at an early age, or if he's an African-American. These are all considerations.

Once the presence of cancer is confirmed, the PSA results can be used to estimate the approximate extent of the disease. The higher the PSA the more likely it is that the tumor is large and the cancer has extended beyond the prostate. Again, there are exceptions. Some patients with a high PSA may have small, curable cancers. Some men with a low PSA may have more advanced disease. Even with the exceptions and inaccuracies, the PSA test remains the most valuable tool available for diagnosing and monitoring prostate cancer.

The most important factor in deciding on treatment is whether or not the cancer has *metastasized*, that is, spread to parts of the body beyond the prostate. The

Table 2

Other Factors that Affect PSA Levels

- Benign prostatic hypertrophy (BPH)
- Infection (prostatitis)
- Trauma such as biopsy or overly vigorous digital rectal examination *(DRE)*
- Ejaculation (a 40 percent elevation, returning to normal within 48 hours)
- Strenuous exercise involving the buttocks or perineum (such as bicycle riding)
- Medical procedures such as balloon dilation of the prostate, transrectal ultrasound-guided biopsy, and transurethral resection of the prostate (TURP)
- Medications such as finasteride (Proscar or Propecia) used to treat BPH can decrease PSA levels by as much as 50 percent.
- Some herbal mixtures marked "for prostate health" may also affect PSA levels.

higher the PSA value, the larger a tumor is likely to be, and the greater the likelihood that the cancer has spread outside the prostate gland. Taken together, the PSA and DRE tests are very useful for detecting cancer, but they provide only rough estimates of how far the disease has actually progressed. As discussed below, more tests are necessary to determine the precise stage and grade of the disease. Staging and grading are standard systems for classifying the disease, that is, for evaluating the nature or grade of the malignancy, and the extent of the disease. All of this information is critical for deciding which treatment options are available for each patient.

Before having a biopsy, you should have your PSA tested several times at the same laboratory. There can be considerable variation with PSA test results depending on the lab and the particular test used. The FDA has approved a number of PSA tests, or assays, produced by various manufacturers; however, many of these tests have been approved only for PSA monitoring, not for diagnosis. Test results can vary by as much as 8 to 10 percent even when the test is done by the same laboratory. This variation is not considered significant, but it is important for patients to try to have their annual PSA test performed by the same lab each year, or at least to use the same FDA-approved brand of test.

Patients are advised to check with their local laboratory to find out what brand of test is being used. You will want to be sure that the particular test at your lab has been FDA-approved for *both* diagnosis and monitoring of prostate cancer.

Why is there Controversy about PSA Screening?

Critics of PSA screening contend that the test detects many incidental, non-aggressive cancers that don't need to be diagnosed or treated because such cancers will never become life-threatening for the patient. The critics argue that many patients are being tested and treated unnecessarily. They also question whether curative treatments for prostate cancer improve survival, even though the most recent studies do indicate that screening and treatment significantly reduce prostate cancer mortality (see the studies cited in Appendix A).

At a meeting of the American Society for Therapeutic Radiology and Oncology (ASTRO) in October 2005, researchers from Brigham and Women's Hospital and the Dana-Farber Cancer Institute reported that annual PSA screening dramatically reduced the risk of dying from prostate cancer. In a retrospective study of 1,492 prostate cancer patients, those who had not had yearly screening tests were three times more likely to die of prostate cancer over the next 10 years than men who received an annual PSA test. This study also showed that even with patients who failed initial treatment, there was still a survival benefit in having been diagnosed with an earlier-stage disease.

Much of the continuing controversy centers on the long-term medical value of PSA screening and its cost-effectiveness. Critics are correct in pointing out that due to its sensitivity, the PSA reports a significant percentage of "false positives," though at our institution we are finding less than 10 percent of men with PSA readings over 10 do not have cancer. Some of these men will suffer the anxiety, inconvenience, and expense of further testing in order to rule out prostate cancer.

We believe that early testing can save many lives, and therefore, the cost and inconvenience appear to be justified. While the mortality rate for prostate cancer in Western nations has been declining since about 1992, according to American Cancer Society estimates, more than 191,930 American men will be newly diagnosed with prostate cancer by the end of 2020, and approximately 33,330 men will die of the disease.

Critics argue that as many as 30 percent of men over the age of 50 have cancers that are insignificant, that will grow slowly and never cause any problem during their lifetimes. This estimate is based on the National Cancer Institute's 2002

Surveillance, Epidemiology and End Results (SEER) data. According to this argument, there is no point in diagnosing or treating these cancers. But a number of studies have shown that most prostate cancers diagnosed with PSA testing are clinically significant and potentially life-threatening. In a study conducted on men who were autopsied, no patient with a PSA greater than 4 had cancer that was clinically incidental. Moreover, in some men who appear to have incidental cancers, the disease will develop later, and they may eventually die of their cancer.

Although doctors have a difficult time distinguishing between cancers that are aggressive and those that are clinically insignificant, the fact remains that most prostate cancers are potentially life-threatening. Once prostate cancer is diagnosed, doctors have a responsibility to make their patients aware of their treatment options and the risks involved. A number of studies have shown that the overall impact on survival has been improved with screening and treatment, and researchers have compiled extensive data (based on PSA monitoring and prostate biopsy) to ascertain cure rates for each treatment modality.

It stands to reason that the only way the large number of annual prostate cancer deaths is likely to be reduced is with early detection and treatment. As of 2020, in the U.S., the death rate from prostate cancer has dropped approximately one-third since the mid-1990s, and much of that improvement is likely the result of screening and improved treatment techniques. The use of PSA-related screening techniques moves up diagnosis of the disease by 5 to 10 years. Such early detection regimens shift the stage at the time of detection towards locally confined disease, and there is no doubt that early treatment is the most effective way of curing prostate cancer.

With that said, it should be emphasized that every man must make his own personal choice on whether to be tested for prostate cancer; and those patients who are diagnosed with the disease have the right to make the decision of whether or not to be treated. While there is no single treatment or set of answers for all patients, each man can make informed decisions about diagnosis and treatment.

What is PSA Velocity?

PSA velocity refers to the rate of change of the PSA over time. The measurement of PSA velocity is known as PSAV or PSA slope. The assumption is that the annual rate of change of the PSA value for men with cancer is greater than the rate of change for men without cancer, including both those with normal prostate glands and those with BPH. A rise in the PSA of 0.75 or more in a year may be an indicator of cancer. A rise in the PSA less than 0.75 might indicate BPH, or could be a fluctuation attributed to a normal prostate.

Studies have shown that the use of PSA velocity can reduce the number of unnecessary biopsies. For patients with BPH and not cancer, PSA velocity may significantly reduce the number of biopsies. PSA velocity can be especially telling for patients whose PSA is within the normal range but increasing rapidly. For example, a patient whose PSA rises from 1.3 to 2.3 to 3.7 over a period of two years might have a cancer detectable with a biopsy even before his PSA climbs above the normal limit of 4.0. This is where the benefit of early detection becomes most obvious, as the cancer can be caught when it is most treatable.

PSA velocity is also useful in diagnosing those patients whose PSA values are in the grey area between 4 and 10, and who have negative biopsies. For example, a patient with a 5.8 PSA value and negative biopsy might undergo another biopsy the next year if his PSA climbs significantly. An increase in PSA of less than 0.75 may rule out the need for another biopsy. The measurement of the PSA values over time greatly increases the ability of a doctor to make an accurate clinical diagnosis. For best results, the patient is usually advised to have his PSA tested at least three times over a period of two years.

While the PSA test can be very important, and may be the single most important marker to determine the likelihood of cancer being present, the PSA alone may not be as important as the PSA velocity. The history of a patient's PSA over time also enables us to obtain the doubling time (PSADT)—the amount of time it takes for the PSA value to double—which can help us determine how rapidly the cancer is growing. A PSADT of less than 12 years and a PSA velocity greater than 0.75 indicate greater likelihood of malignancy.

What are Free and Bound PSA?

Several other approaches for measuring PSA levels can allow us to make a more accurate diagnosis. Among these are free (or unbound) versus bound (or complexed) PSA. These terms refer to the fact that PSA appears in the bloodstream in two distinct molecular forms, either unattached to other substances (free), or combined with other protein molecules (bound). The *percent-free PSA test* measures how much free PSA circulates in the bloodstream compared to the total PSA level. The percentage of free PSA tends to be lower in men who have prostate cancer than in men who do not.

Some studies indicate that the amount of bound PSA in the blood is higher when cancer is present, while the amount of free PSA is higher in men with BPH. The percent-free PSA test is especially useful for diagnosing patients whose PSA falls into the grey area between 4 and 10, and even at lower levels between 2.5 and 4 —when it is most difficult to distinguish cancer from benign enlargement of the prostate (BPH). By increasing the accuracy of PSA testing in this way, the number of unnecessary biopsies can be reduced.

The free PSA test is more specific than total PSA by itself. This means that fewer patients without cancer test false positive. Because the percent-free PSA threshold of less than 25% is more specific for a diagnosis of cancer, it avoids the need for biopsy in about 20% of patients who would otherwise undergo this procedure based upon total PSA alone. The percent-free PSA test can also be a valuable asset for monitoring patients after treatment.

What is PSA Density?

Another way we can sometimes distinguish between cancer and BPH is by measuring the PSA density, which is the PSA value divided by the volume of the prostate gland, as determined by transrectal ultrasound. For a man with an enlarged prostate, the PSA value should not be greater than 15% of the weight of the prostate. Anything higher than that may be indicative of prostate cancer. The measurement of PSA density can help determine which men with slightly elevated PSA values should be subjected to biopsies to confirm or rule out the presence of cancer.

What is the PAP Test?

At our institution, a PAP (Prostatic Acid Phosphatase) blood test is also routinely performed, as this test has been demonstrated by our team as well as other researchers in the medical literature to be perhaps the single most adverse feature associated with prostate cancer. Before the advent of the PSA test, the PAP test was the only prostate tumor marker. In fact, doctors believed that the test was so accurate that if the patient had an elevated PAP, he should not undergo surgery because he would predictably have cancer outside the prostate gland, and therefore could not be cured by surgery.

After the advent of the PSA test, the PAP became less and less used. However, we never stopped using it and have even found that this test can be an independent prognosticator for treatment failure. In other words, in patients undergoing radiation therapy, we found that the PAP was as important as the PSA, and possibly more important for patients with advanced cancer, so we routinely employ it (See Taira A, Merrick G, Wallner K, Dattoli M. Reviving the acid phosphatase test for prostate cancer, Oncology Williston Park. 2007 Jul;21(8):1003-10 and Fang LC, Dattoli M, Taira A, True L, Sorace R, Wallner K. Prostatic acid phosphatase adversely affects cause-specific survival Urology. 2008 Jan;71(1):146-50).

Similar to radiation data, the PAP also carries tremendous statistical power for predicting whether or not a patient will relapse after surgery. Recent studies are finding that in patients with an elevated PAP, over 85% of those patients are going to fail after surgery. This should be no surprise in view of older pre-PSA surgical data. The PAP test is a solid-phase chemiluminescent immunometric assay. The normal reference range for a healthy male is < 3.5ng/ml.

Table 3
Factors That Can Cause Abnormal PAP Values

- Prostate cancer, especially prostate cancer that has spread outside the prostate
- Infection (prostatitis)
- Decreased blood flow to the prostate
- Paget's disease (bones become thicker and softer)
- Anemia
- Thrombophlebitis
- Gaucher's disease
- Hyperparathyroidism
- Heart attack
- Kidney disease
- Physical stimulation of the prostate (colonoscopy, enemas, prostate examination)
- Multiple myeloma

What is the PCA3Plus™ Test?

PCA3Plus™ is a urine-based genetic test for prostate cancer risk. This test detects PCA3, a specific gene that is highly expressed in prostate cancer. In fact, no other human tissues express PCA3.

This test is the second generation of another highly successful test known as uPM3™. PCA3Plus™ tests for prostate cancer cells that are shed into the urine (following a digital rectal exam). The urine sample is sent to a laboratory to be tested for genetic expression of the PCA3 gene. If the sample tests positive for PCA3, then the patient has a very high likelihood of having prostate cancer. PCA3Plus™, when validated, predicts prostate cancer with a sensitivity of 95.7%.

One advantage of the PCA3Plus™ genetic test is that it can help reduce the number of prostate biopsies based on PSA and DRE tests (see below, "What is a Prostate Biopsy?"). According to researchers at the Johns Hopkins University School of Medicine, due to elevated PSA levels, approximately 1.6 million men undergo prostatic biopsies in the U.S. each year, and roughly 80% of these men end up having negative results. As doctors continue to add to their arsenal of diagnostic workup tests, early detection of the disease becomes more accurate and reliable, reducing the number of unnecessary biopsies.

What is a Prostate Biopsy and How is it Performed?

A prostate biopsy is a procedure by which samples of tissue are removed from suspicious areas of the prostate gland for microscopic examination by a pathologist. **A biopsy is absolutely necessary to confirm the presence of cancer** and should be undertaken prior to any treatment of the disease. The biopsy also provides us with a wealth of information about the specific characteristics of the cancer.

When performing a biopsy, the doctor will use an imaging technique called transrectal ultrasound (TRUS) for guidance in order to insert a narrow needle through the wall of the rectum into the prostate gland (see below "What is Transrectal Ultrasound (TRUS)? In recent years, ultrasound-guided biopsies are often performed with additional guidance provided by magnetic resonance imaging (MRI). This advanced imaging technique allows for more precise targeting of the biopsy needles to remove tissue samples from the prostate (see below, "What is the Multiparametric MRI?").

At our institution, we perform the biopsy through the perineum, the area between the rectum and scrotum. This is known as a transperineal biopsy. The needle removes a tiny core of tissue (usually measuring about 1/2-inch by 1/16-inch) that is sent to the laboratory to see if cancer is present. Although the procedure may sound painful, for most men, a biopsy causes little discomfort because it is performed with an instrument called a biopsy gun which inserts and removes the needle in a fraction of a second. In addition, a local anesthetic can be used to numb the area. Patients are advised to confirm this with their doctor prior to the procedure. The procedure can be done in the doctor's office and usually takes only about 15 minutes.

The prostate biopsy has traditionally involved obtaining at least six core samples of tissue. This procedure, known as the sextant biopsy, draws two tissue samples from the base, mid-gland and apex for a total of six core samples. Studies have shown that increasing the number of samples can significantly increase the detection of malignancy. The number of biopsy samples taken now typically ranges from 6 to 18 or more. The 5-region biopsy approach obtains additional samples from the mid-gland tissue and the lateral zones or lobes on each side of the gland. When a very large number of samples are obtained (30 samples or more), this approach is called "saturation biopsy."

Your biopsy report should indicate how many tissue samples were taken from specific areas of the prostate, and how many specimens showed cancer (see below, "How Are Biopsy Results Reported?"). The report should also indicate what percentage of each core contained cancer and how many specimens showed solid cores. If each core is solid, then the tumor is likely to be large. If the cores are small and scattered, the needle probably passed through small tumors. More than 50% cancer in any one core and/or multiple positive cores would suggest a larger tumor. When more than half of a prostate lobe is involved, the outlook is less optimistic because larger tumors have a less favorable prognosis.

Your doctor will use all of this information about the size and extent of your cancer, along with the results of the rest of the workup tests, to develop a strategy for treating the disease. Recent studies have shown that biopsies guided by the Color-Flow Power Doppler Ultrasound imaging technique have the advantage of showing the optimal sites from which to secure tissue samples.

Once the initial diagnosis has been established, we request that the specimen slides be reviewed by a pathologist who specializes in prostate pathology. Specialists in evaluating prostate biopsy specimens are available at a number of labs and major medical centers. Samples can be sent to these specialists for "second opinions," as the pathological interpretation can vary. There is an "art" to interpreting the slides, and it is that interpretation that your doctor will use in helping you to determine how to best treat the disease.

With respect to saturation biopsies, at our center we perform them for both practical and theoretical reasons. The procedure is commonly referred to as "template-guided transperineal 3-dimensional mapping (3-DMP)." This technique is virtually the same as performing brachytherapy (radioactive seed implantation) from the standpoint of patient positioning (dorso-lithotomy), using a regional anesthetic, and using the brachytherapy template grid. The only real difference is that seeds are not deposited but rather tissue is extracted using a biopsy gun.

This approach to biopsy avoids some of the limitations associated with the standard transrectal approach. These include the ability to better access and sample the apical prostate (lowest portion), anterior prostate (transitional zone) and the most postero-lateral (left and right) aspects of the gland, all of which can be challenging and sometimes simply not possible with the standard transrectal method (especially in larger glands).

The risk of infection is less with the 3-DMP approach as is the degree of rectal bleeding, since the rectal wall is not pierced, while only a betadine cleansed "sterile" perineum is pierced using the 3-DMP method. Its only drawback is that it is much more costly. Since the rectum is spared entirely, there is no risk of bleeding or contamination that might cause infection.

At our center, we have a policy to perform the 3-DMP method only as a follow-up approach to one or two negative sets of standard in-office biopsies OR in cases where it is clear that the abnormal area(s) of color flow perfusion is(are) outside of where we feel we can reach with the biopsy gun using the standard technique. One additional advantage to the 3-DMP method is that it may better determine which cases can be theoretically managed with "expectant management" or "active surveillance," which involve patients having "insignificant cancer," since the likelihood of "undersampling of the disease" is very small (Carter HB, et al, *J Urol*, 2002, 167::1231-1234).

Dr. Dattoli on Anesthetic Techniques Utilized for Painless Prostate Biopsies

At our center, in order to provide our patients with prostate biopsies that are as painless as possible, we may utilize a combination of Periprostatic Nerve Block (PNB) and Pelvic Plexus Block (PPB) local anesthetic techniques coupled with mild sedation. The biopsy procedure is initiated with an intravenous (IV) injection of propofol, which causes sedation. Following the injection, the PNB and PPB anesthetic techniques can be used to minimize discomfort after a patient undergoes an Image-Guided Transperineal Prostate Biopsy, when core samples are obtained through a needle template similar to that used for brachytherapy seed implantation.

Both the PNB and PPB procedures are performed in conjunction with 3D Color-Flow Power Doppler Ultrasound and MRI imaging guidance. For the Periprostatic Nerve Block, lidocaine solution is injected into the neurovascular bundles at the juncture of the prostate, bladder and seminal vesicle. For the Pelvic Plexus Block, lidocaine injections are administered to the pelvic neurovascular plexus, located at the end of and just lateral to the seminal vesicles.

Core samples are typically removed bilaterally from the prostate base, mid-zone, and apex. These anesthetic techniques complement each other such that the transperineal biopsy procedure is virtually painless for our patients. On a pain scale of 0 to 10, none of our patients report any discomfort greater than 1.

What is the Gleason Score?

Under the microscope, prostate cancer cells exhibit a particular range of aggressiveness, from slow-growing to fast-growing, and they are ranked accordingly. The ranking used to identify how aggressive or abnormal a cancer appears is called the Gleason scale. The scale essentially runs from 2 to 10, with the least aggressive tumors at the low end and the fastest growing, more aggressive tumors at the high end of the scale.

Slow-growing tumors appear similar to normal tissue and are called "well-differentiated." Fast-growing cancers appear abnormal and are called "poorly differentiated." Between the two extremes are cancers which are classified as moderately differentiated." The Gleason system defines five glandular patterns of cancerous cell tissue, from completely differentiated to completely undifferentiated.

Tumors often possess more than one cellular pattern in different tissue samples, and therefore, both primary and secondary patterns are graded. The two grades are combined (added together) to get the actual Gleason score, ranging from 2 (1+1) to 10 (5+5), with most cancers falling somewhere in between (see Figure 2). The higher the Gleason score, the more likely it is that the cancer is more aggressive and has already spread beyond the prostate capsule or metastasized to other parts of the body.

Unfortunately, like the PSA scale, the Gleason scale provides only an approximation of how aggressive a cancer is and how likely it is that the cancer has spread.

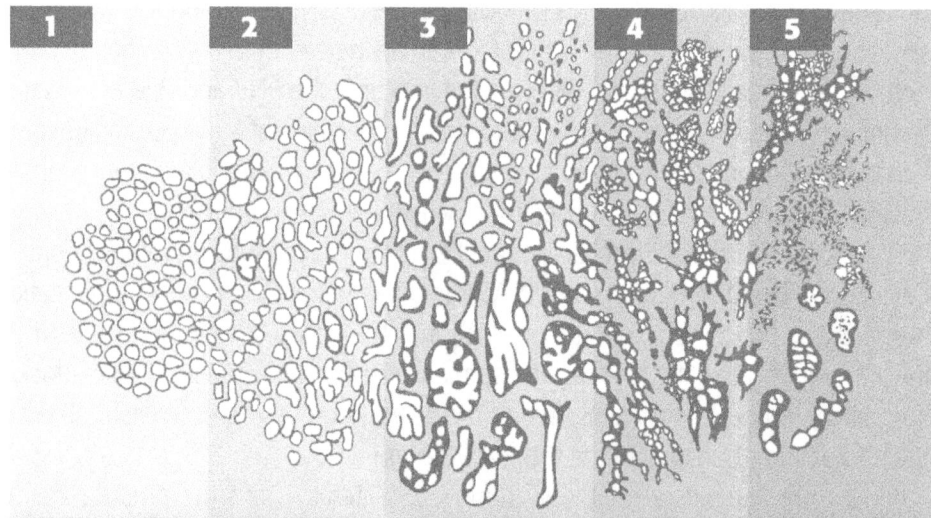

Figure 2—A simplified drawing of the Gleason grading system, showing the five distinct grades of cancerous tissue, as seen under low magnification. The two most common cell patterns seen in the tissue sample are added together to arrive at a Gleason score.

One part of the prostate gland may appear to be more aggressive or abnormal than other parts, and there is some element of chance as to where exactly the biopsy needles obtains each specimen. The imprecision of Gleason scoring creates exceptions when interpreting the numbers. Some men with high Gleason scores may have small, curable cancers, while other men with lower numbers may have cancers that are more advanced. Nevertheless, the Gleason score is fairly accurate in predicting how aggressive the cancer is and how rapidly it will spread.

What is DNA Ploidy Analysis?

Another test sometimes performed by the pathologist utilizes a hi-tech examination called flow cytometry to analyze the nuclear DNA content, or DNA Ploidy, of cancer cells. Samples for analysis may be obtained from biopsy or operating tissue. The genetic information derived from this test allows cancer cells to be classified as "diploid," "tetraploid," or "aneuploid." Aneuploid cancers generally have a less favorable prognosis than diploid cancers, and if left untreated are more likely to progress rapidly. Diploid cancers have a more favorable prognosis than either aneuploid or tetraploid. Why ploidies differ and why some indicate a more aggressive cancer than others remains the subject of continuing research.

While this method of analysis is very sensitive, the predictive value of flow cytometry is not definitive, and the test is not reliable enough to be used by itself as a diagnostic tool. As far as determining the aggressiveness of the tumor, ploidy can be enhanced when combined with the patient's PSA and Gleason score. It is a subject of debate whether the data on ploidy is solid enough to be used as a basis for treatment decisions. Most physicians do not rely on this form of testing and consider it investigational or supplemental in light of other test results. When ploidy is used, it is most often called for when the patient's Gleason score is greater than or equal to 7. Some studies have suggested that if the PSA is greater than or equal to 15, and if the ploidy is aneuploid, then the likelihood is that the cancer will already have metastasized.

How are Biopsy Results Reported?

Aside from the grade of the cancer (when present), the pathologist's report often contains other pieces of information that may give a better idea of the extent of the cancer. These can include: 1) the number of biopsy core samples that contain cancer—for example, "6 out of 12", 2) the percentage of cancer in each of the cores, and 3) whether the cancer is on the left side or right side or both sides of the prostate.

Sometimes when the pathologist examines the prostate cells under the microscope, they don't look cancerous, and yet they don't appear to be normal. These results are often reported as "suspicious." Suspicious results generally fall into two categories—either "prostatic intraepithelial neoplasia" (PIN) or "atypical small acinar proliferation" (ASAP).

In the case of PIN, there are changes in how the prostate cells appear under the microscope, but the cells are basically still in place. Unlike cancer cells, they don't appear to have invaded into other parts of the prostate. PIN is often divided into low-grade and-high grade. Many men begin to develop low-grade PIN at an early age and will not necessarily develop prostate cancer.

If high-grade PIN is found, there is about a 20% chance that cancer may already be present somewhere else in the prostate gland. For this reason, doctors often watch men with high-grade PIN carefully and may advise a repeat prostate biopsy, especially if the original biopsy did not take samples from all parts of the prostate.

In the case of ASAP, also called atypia, the prostate cells look like they might be cancerous when examined under the microscope, but there are too few of these cells to be certain. When ASAP is present, there is approximately a 40% to 50% chance that cancer is also present in the prostate, which is why many doctors recommend getting a repeat biopsy within a few months.

Laboratory pathology reports vary a great deal from laboratory to laboratory, and they can be difficult for patients without medical training to interpret. You may need to consult with your physician to gain a full understanding of what the reports reveal about your individual diagnostic condition. Nevertheless, you should be able to identify a number of important pieces of information about your case, depending on which tests you have undergone.

The various lab reports can inform you about the basic status of your condition, your PSA level, your Gleason score, your DNA ploidy analysis, the size of the tumor and how far it has spread, and the stage of the cancer. The biopsy report usually contains a Case Summary and a Gross Description of the size, location and number of tissue samples obtained. It will also contain a technical Microscopic Description, often filled with complicated technical information about the cellular characteristics of the tumor, such as the architecture and polarity of the cells. Patients are well advised to discuss these specific details of their biopsy reports with their doctors.

What is Transrectal Ultrasound (TRUS)?

Technically referred to a transrectal ultrasonography, this is a technique that projects sound waves off the prostate and surrounding organs to create an image. The sound waves are generated by a probe placed inside the rectum. Transrectal ultrasound imaging can in many cases accurately identify the local spread of cancer outside the prostate gland. In some cases, however, areas of cancer growth outside the prostate gland may be too small to be visible. As mentioned, ultrasound is often used to guide the biopsy needle to suspicious sites in the prostate. The technique is also used for real time guidance in conjunction with seed implants, external radiation therapy, and other treatments. At our institution, Color-Flow Power Doppler Ultrasound (CFPDU) is utilized since it provides enhanced visualization and greater definition compared to the conventional gray-scale. The Color-Flow Power Doppler Ultrasound imaging technique improves the likelihood of obtaining biopsy needle samples from potential tumor sites.

While there is an art to interpreting Color-Flow Power Doppler images, tumors tend to demonstrate increased blood perfusion or hypervascularity as findings consistent with malignancy. Tumors grow faster than normal prostate cells and require more blood to nurture their growth. Tumors therefore tend to create blood vessels around them as they grow, and these can be identified by Color-Flow Power Doppler Ultrasound. A conventional TRUS typically shows what are called hypoechogenic areas, which are darker shades of gray. A Color-Flow Power Doppler Ultrasound may show the same image, but it provides additional insight into how much perfusion of blood is going into the region, and can reveal whether just one prostate nodule is involved or if there is more cancer dispersed throughout the gland.

What are CT Scans and Fused Imaging Modalities?

The CT scan (also called CAT scan) uses computer tomography to produce a 3-dimensional image of the prostate and surrounding organs. CT scans rely on computer-reconstructed x-rays to give a cross-sectional view of the body. A CT scan through the pelvis reveals the outline of the prostate. CT scans can identify prostate enlargement and show the size and shape of the gland, but it is not as effective for assessing the extent of cancer or visualizing cancer within the gland itself. While CT scans provide less defined images of the outer prostatic contour and internal architecture, CT images do accurately delineate the spatial relationship between the prostate, rectum and pubic bones. More contemporary spiral or helical CT scans provide greater resolution while taking less time to acquire the information.

The circular track magnet of the CT scanner directs pinpoint-thin x-ray beams through the portions of the body under examination as it rapidly passes over the patient. Each pass of the CT scanner provides a cross-section of the body's internal structures, and as many as eight scans per centimeter are taken.

The data is fed into a computer, which converts the information into a three-dimensional image. The image gives a more precise and accurate picture of the internal organs than the flat view provided by a conventional x-ray, which superimposes overlapping organs and can only dimly represent the soft tissues of the body.

Today the CT scan is often combined or fused with other sophisticated imaging and diagnostic modalities, such as multiparametric MRI (mpMRI) and Dynamic Contrast Enhanced MRI (DCE-MRI). These fused imaging modalities represent the state of the art in imaging and have greatly enhanced our ability to diagnose and treat the disease.

What is Magnetic Resonance Imaging (MRI) and How Does It Work?

Magnetic resonance imaging (MRI) is an advanced imaging technique that generates a powerful magnetic field, which harmlessly reacts with tissues in the body to produce a distinct and complex image of internal organs. Researchers have been developing MRI for prostate imaging since the 1980s. Technological innovations in recent years have allowed for a more detailed visualization of the gland that aids doctors in detecting and staging prostate cancer.

In the past the MRI was primarily used in staging biopsy-proven prostate cancer. Today, an MRI scan is often performed prior to the ultrasound-guided biopsy to pinpoint the suspicious areas of the gland where the needles will be targeted. With conventional MRI, known as endorectal MRI, a rectal probe is utilized. The probe or coil is similar to a transrectal ultrasound probe. The MRI probe is placed inside the rectum and can allow doctors to image the prostate with enough detail to detect cancer that has spread outside the prostate.

Early MRI machines were equipped with a 1.5 Tesla magnet (1.5T). Tesla refers to the unit of measurement quantifying the strength of the magnetic field. Today we have MRI machines equipped with 3 Tesla magnets. Because the 3T magnet is so powerful, the MRI procedure does not require the invasive endorectal probe that 1.5T MRI machines require. This technique is known as Tesla 3 MRI. The high resolution, 3T MRI images of the prostate look like HDTV. The 3T MRI technique is more accurate than CT scans or standard grey-scale ultrasound for detecting cancer that has spread beyond the prostate.

What are Multiparametric MRI and PI-RADS Analysis?

Multiparametric MRI (mpMRI) involves a sequence of imaging techniques that provide detailed anatomical and functional information that is not possible with grey scale ultrasound. Radiologists can use multiparametric MRI to identify the location of a tumor or tumors, to measure the extent of a tumor, and to determine whether a tumor has spread beyond the prostate gland. Multiparametric MRI scanning usually consists of three distinct imaging techniques (parameters): T2-weighted MRI, diffusion-weighted MRI, and Dynamic Contrast Enhanced MRI (DCE-MRI).

A T2-weighted MRI exam provides doctors with anatomic information about the prostate gland. This technique is useful for the detection, localization and staging of prostate cancers. It offers detailed visualizations of the prostate and its three distinct zones:

- The peripheral zone (PZ) contains the most prostatic tissue. The largest area of the peripheral zone is at the back surface of the gland near the rectal wall. When a doctor performs a digital rectal exam, it is the back of the gland that he is feeling. Approximately 70-80% of prostate cancers originate in the peripheral zone.
- The central zone (CZ) surrounds the ejaculatory ducts. Less than 5% of prostate cancers originate in this zone, and they are often more aggressive and more likely to invade the seminal vesicles.
- The transition zone (TZ) surrounds the urethra where it enters the gland. This area grows in men over the years and is responsible for benign prostatic hyperplasia (BPH). About 20% of prostate cancers originate in this zone.

On T2-weighted MRI images, tumors in the peripheral zone of the prostate typically appear as bright spots against a dark background. Cancers in the transition zone are more difficult to detect. They may appear as smudged charcoal against a dark background. T2-weighted MRI scans are also used to evaluate the seminal vesicles and bladder wall to determine if a tumor has spread beyond the prostate.

Diffusion-weighted imaging (DWI) measures the motion of water molecules within the prostate, which provides useful functional information about cancers. This sequence produces an ADC value for different areas of the prostate gland. ADC values measure the degree of motion through different tissues. Lower ADC values appear in cancerous tissue than in healthy tissue. The ADC values also tend to correlate with Gleason scores, with lower ADC values indicating a higher Gleason score

At our institution, approximately 90% of our patients undergo an MRI prior to treatment, preferably Dynamic Contrast Enhanced MRI, which is superior to any other type of MRI currently available (including the spectroscopic MRI—or MRSI). DCE-MRI provides more detailed imaging than MRSI. With the Dynamic Contrast Enhanced MRI, a contrast agent is administered to the patient and is used to evaluate blood flow through the prostate. Cancerous tissue absorbs the contrast agent more quickly than healthy tissue, which is revealed on DCE images. MRI contrast agents such as Feraheme and Combidex are also being utilized to identify lymph node and bone metastases (for more on this subject, see the Dattoli Cancer Foundation booklet, *Lymph Node Positive Prostate Cancer: Advanced Diagnostics and Treatment*).

Contrast Enhanced MRI is similar to and complements Color-Flow Power Doppler Ultrasound. When cancer is revealed on the DCE-MRI, we will also see it on ultrasound. However, we also sometimes see tumors on Color-Flow Power Doppler TRUS that are missed by MRI scans. Because of the limited view of the prostate gland provided by both MRI and ultrasound imaging, some cancers may be missed on larger glands, those greater than 50 cc. The only reason a patient would not have an MRI in our practice is if his insurance company would not pay for it and the patient can't afford the test, as it is expensive. The cost of a diagnostic pelvic MRI is at least two to three times higher than the cost for a TRUS or CT scan.

Multiparametric MRI studies are interpreted according to the Prostate Imaging Reporting and Data System (PI-RADS, Version 2). This is a classification system that uses a 5-point scale to standardize the evaluation of multiparametric MRI. A PI-RADS interpretation indicates the likelihood of indolent prostate cancer versus clinically significant prostate cancer (intermediate and high-risk cancers) based on the three multiparametric MRI techniques.

PI-RADS 1–Highly unlikely that clinically significant cancer is present.

PI-RADS 2–Unlikely that clinically significant cancer is present.

PI-RADS 3–Uncertain whether clinically significant cancer is present.

PI-RADS 4–Likely that clinically significant cancer is present.

PI-RADS 5–Highly likely that clinically significant cancer is present.

With PI-RADS 4 or 5 results, patients should be recommended for biopsy. For results of PI-RADS 1 or 2, a recommendation for biopsy would likely be inappropriate, though other factors may also be considered. For results of PI-RADS 3, biopsy may be deemed appropriate taking into account a patient's history and preferences in consultation with his physician.

One of the benefits of multiparametric MRI is its ability to help men decide on Active Surveillance (AS) as a management strategy rather than undergoing primary therapies such as radical prostatectomy or radiation therapy. Monitoring men in Active Surveillance was previously accomplished using only evaluations based on

PSA testing and blind biopsy. With multiparametric MRI, doctors are able to better determine which patients are likely to have low-risk, indolent disease rather than intermediate and high-risk disease. This approach allows men with low-risk disease to delay primary therapy and possible side effects, until there is evidence of disease progression (a rising PSA).

Another important benefit of multiparametric MRI is that it allows for targeted biopsies. Biopsy needles can be guided using real-time MRI images or multiparametric MRI images can be fused with real-time ultrasound images to guide biopsy needles. These procedures are referred to as MRI-guided biopsy and MRI-TRUS fusion biopsy respectively. When PI-RADS evaluation is used to triage men for biopsy, both MRI-guided and MRI-TRUS fusion biopsy offer improved diagnostic outcomes with fewer needles compared to the conventional grey-scale ultrasound-guided biopsy.

A PSA screening program that incorporates multiparametric MRI is likely to improve screening for prostate cancer in a number of ways:

- By reducing the total number of biopsies and total number of biopsy needles used, reducing complications associated with biopsy.
- By improving the diagnostic accuracy for intermediate- and high-risk prostate cancers.
- By more accurately improving the detection of low-risk, indolent prostate cancers.
- By more accurately recommending Active Surveillance for low-risk patients when appropriate rather than primary treatment.

Once prostate cancer is confirmed by biopsy, that detailed anatomic and functional information provided by multiparametric MRI can help to guide treatment decisions. For instance, multiparametric MRI can effectively identify seminal vesicle invasion, extraprostatic extension and pelvic lymph node involvement.

Patients considering multiparametric MRI are advised to take into account the technology used by different radiology facilities and the experience (or lack of experience) of radiologists interpreting scans. Many studies suggest that multiparametric MRI is more effectively performed with 3T MRI machines. In addition, studies suggest that multiparametric MRI exams are more accurately interpreted by radiologists with extensive experience evaluating these advanced imaging techniques.

A 2014 multinational study compared conventional gray-scale ultrasound-guided biopsies with multiparametric MRI-targeted biopsies with PI-RADS interpretation. Researchers reported the following improved results with multiparametric MRI with PI-RADS:

51% reduction in number of biopsies compared with TRUS.

84% reduction in number of biopsy needles used.

89.4% reduction in detection of low-risk, indolent cancer.

17.7% increase in detection of intermediate- and high-risk cancer.

By using multiparametric MRI and PI-RADS interpretation to selectively guide biopsies in patients with elevated PSA, instead of conventional ultrasound-guided biopsy, this study showed a reduction in the need for biopsy while improving overall detection of clinically significant intermediate and high-risk cancers (Pokorny MR, et al, Eur Urol. 2014 Jul;66(1):22-9).

A 2015 study published by researchers at the National Cancer Institute showed even greater improvement with MRI-TRUS fusion-guided biopsies. These researchers reported a reduction of 17% in the detection of low-risk cancers with an increase of 30% in the detection of high risk cancers compared to conventional TRUS-guided biopsies. This study demonstrated that MRI-TRUS fusion biopsy was associated with an increase in the detection of intermediate and high-risk prostate cancers and decreased detection of low-risk, indolent prostate cancers (Okoro C, et al, J Endourol. 2015 Oct;29(10):1115-21).

In addition to reducing the number of biopsies, image-guided biopsies that utilize both the Color-Flow Power Doppler Ultrasound and multiparametric MRI techniques can save lives by improving the efficacy of PSA screening. The bottom line is that doctors utilizing these imaging modalities are better able to determine which patients are not at risk for clinically significant prostate cancer and do not need to undergo biopsies. Some of these low-risk patients may elect to pursue Active Surveillance rather than undergo an aggressive primary treatment such a surgery or radiation.

A recent long term study by the Memorial Sloan Kettering Cancer Center suggests that many patients who pursue Active Surveillance are only postponing treatment. For select, low risk patients on AS, the likelihood of avoiding treatment at 5, 10, and 15 years was 76%, 64%, and 58% respectively (Carisson S, et al, J Urol, 2019, Dec 23).

Dattoli Team Biopsy Results with Color-Flow Power Doppler Ultrasound

When doing biopsies at our center, in order to guide the biopsy needles to take samples from the prostate, as mentioned, we use both the conventional grayscale ultrasound and 3D Color-Flow Power Doppler Ultrasound (3D-CFPDU). Most patients at other medical centers are biopsied using only the grayscale ultrasound, which is a piece of technology that costs about $40,000, whereas the 3D-CFPDU equipment costs many times that. The high cost is one of the reasons this technology is not yet widely available for prostate cancer patients.

With grayscale ultrasound guidance, standard biopsies randomly sample 10 to 12 cores. And we have seen patients with rising PSAs who come to us after having been biopsied elsewhere for several years with negative results. When they come to our center for 3D-CFPDU guided biopsies, it is not uncommon for us to find 10 to 12 positive cores because the Color-Flow Power Doppler technology is far more discerning than grayscale ultrasound. We have demonstrated that with our own studies.

On February 26th, 2015 in Orlando, Florida, at the annual national Genitourinary Cancers Symposium sponsored by the American Society of Clinical Oncology, we presented a study on prostate biopsies using both grayscale and 3-Dimensional Color-Flow Power Doppler Ultrasound.

To summarize our results, we showed that the standard grayscale ultrasound biopsies often lead to sampling errors with mixed diagnosis, delayed diagnosis and the need for repeated biopsies, under-staging, and finding indolent (very slow growing) prostate cancers that often leads to over-treatment. We also pointed out in our study that infections are common with the standard biopsy. The standard approach is to perform the biopsy through the rectal wall, and that approach carries the risk of introducing rectal flora into the bloodstream. That can lead to sepsis, which is a systemic infection, and many patients end up requiring hospitalization when that occurs.

But we reduce the risk of infection and avoid that by using a sterile, transperineal approach to biopsies that is similar to the way we perform brachytherapy seed implants. And our patients are under anesthesia for this procedure. Instead of entering through the rectum with needles, we enter through the perineum, which as noted is the area between the scrotum and anus. We also extend the patient's legs to the dorso-lithotomy position, which gives us much greater access to the prostate. With the standard biopsy, the patient is on his side and the physician is limited by having to go through the rectum with a biopsy gun and is thus unable to sample the entire gland. This is especially limiting with patients who have large glands. With the extended dorso-lithotomy position that we use, the patient is supine with the pelvic arch open so we can more easily take our needle samples directly from the prostate, and we have access to the entire gland even with patients who have enlarged glands due to BPH.

One other advantage of using the transperineal approach is that we know exactly where each core sample comes from, because each needle enters through a template that precisely allows us map the position. Once we have the pathology results, we will know exactly where the cancer is located and can carry out treatments as needed with DART and brachytherapy with great accuracy.

Our 2015 study followed 192 patients, and we divided them into four groups. All but two of the patients had been biopsied previously using grayscale ultrasound. The first group of patients was termed hypoechoic, meaning the visible lesion was seen as a dark area in the ultrasound image. A second group was hypervascular, meaning the lesion was colorful in the image. A third group was hypoechoic with hypervascular pulsatile vessels, meaning the lesion was dark but there was a heart rhythm associated with the blood flow that we could see in the image. And a fourth group was characterized as hypoechoic with non-pulsatile vessels, meaning a dark lesion that is not in sync with the patient's heart. That is because those lesions are growing independently.

The results reported show that for Groups 1 and 2, the biopsy indicated cancer in about 20% of patients, while Group 3 showed 55% positive biopsy results. But Group 4 came back with 97% positive results, with Glesaon scores 7 to 10.

We concluded that transperineal template-guided biopsies using combined grayscale and 3D Color-Flow Power Doppler Ultrasound are highly effective and also cost-effective in a high volume setting by reducing the number of biopsies and enhancing the detection of serious prostate cancers.

What is a Bone Scan?

A bone scan is an imaging technique used to detect bone metastases, which appear as "hot spots" on film. It is far more sensitive than conventional x-rays. The bone scan procedure is performed by injecting a small amount of radioactive dye called technetium into the patient's bloodstream. A special camera is then used to photograph the skeleton, and any irritation of the bone will show up as a spot on the image.

If a patient's PSA is high, greater than 10, or if the Gleason score is greater than or equal to 7, we typically recommend a bone scan. A spot on a bone scan may be caused by cancer that has metastasized, or by arthritis and other causes. When an abnormality shows up on a bone scan, further tests such as traditional x-rays or a CT scan may be used to determine if the cause is cancer. It is important to establish a baseline to differentiate between cancer and other abnormalities.

What are the ProstaVysion and QuadVysion™ Tests?

ProstaVysion is a state-of-the-art diagnostic test that we include in the workup profile for each new patient at the Dattoli Cancer Center. Developed by Bostwick's leading pathology specialists, this multifaceted test is extremely valuable for evaluating how aggressive the cancer is and the likelihood of recurrence after treatment. The ProstaVysion analysis involves a tissue-based, genetic panel. The pathologist utilizes three biomarkers for analysis: HOXD3, ERG and PTEN. By evaluating these three markers, ProstaVysion is able to provide doctors with molecular analysis of the aggressiveness of each patient's cancer and his prognosis, prior to initial primary treatment or salvage therapy.

HOXD3 is one of the genes that regulates cell differentiation and HOXD3 methylation (the modification of a strand of DNA after it is replicated in the cells) is elevated in prostate cancer tissue.

ERG gene fusions (these are hybrid genes formed from two previously separated genes) are found in approximately 40% of primary tumors and suggest a more aggressive cancer. This finding correlates with stage and Gleason score and is predictive of survival rates.

PTEN is a significant tumor suppressor gene in prostate cancer. When the cancer is localized, depletion of PTEN occurs in 20-40% of cases. When the cancer has metastasized, depletion of PTEN is found in 60% of patients with advanced disease.

Each of the three markers provides crucial prognostic information that enables doctors to determine the appropriate course of therapy. Peer-reviewed references and data for each of the three biomarkers are available at the Bostwick Laboratories website: https://www.bostwicklaboratories.com/global/services/laboratory-services/urologic-pathology/prostavysion.aspx.

Bostwick Laboratories also offers the QuadVysion™ immunohistochemistry stain to improve the detection sensitivity for prostate cancer on difficult prostate needle biopsies. The immunohistochemistry stain consists of four antibodies: racemase (P504S), high molecular weight cytokeratin (34ß-E12), p63 and c-myc.

A number of other biomarkers are used to determine the aggressiveness of cancer. These include the following:

Proliferating Cell Nuclear Antigen (PCNA) High PCNA labeling indices may indicate progression of prostate cancer, and may be an independent prognostic indicator.

Ki-67 and MIB-1 Recognizes a nuclear antigen present in proliferating cells but absent in resting cells. Ki-67 labeling index may discriminate between organ confined and metastatic cancer.

Microvessel Density (MVD) This measurement is helpful in predicting pathologic stage and patient outcome in prostate cancer.

Bcl-2

- Highlights the Bcl-2 protein which functions as a blocker of apoptosis and programmed cell death.

- Expression of Bcl-2 is normally restricted to the basal cell layer of the normal and hyperplastic prostatic epithelium.
- Overexpression of Bcl-2 is present in high-grade prostatic intraepithelial neoplasia.

p53
- Identifies p53 (a regulator of the cell cycle) immunoreactivity in cancer cells.
- A number of immunohistochemical studies concluded that mutant p53 expression is a late event in localized prostate cancer, usually present in higher (>7) grade cancer.

pP27
- The cyclin-dependent kinase inhibitor (p27Kip1) negatively regulates cell proliferation.
- Decreased p27Kip1 expression may be an independent predictor for cancer recurrence and long-term survival of prostate cancer.

Another diagnostic and predictive biomarker utilizes prostate specific membrane antigen (PSMA). The PSMA-PET imaging technique uses small molecules that bind to PSMA, localizes a prostate cancer tumor, and allows radiologists to detect small sites of disease such as lymph node metastases. This imaging technique is especially useful in detecting oligometastatic disease, which involves a limited number of metastases.

At our center, we employ multiple laboratory tests for genomic and genetic makeup that allow us to determine which specific medications and treatments may be most appropriate for each patient. We utilize both the Invitae Genetic Test and the Myriad myRisk® Hereditary Cancer testing. The Myriad test is a 35-gene panel that identifies elevated risk for eight hereditary cancers. There are a host of genetic pathways and mutations that a patient may have (including BRACA 2, BRCA1, HOXB13, ATM, CHEK2, and CDK1), and they can tell us whether or not a patient is likely to respond well to a particular agent. For example, we know that a patient with positive BRCA1 and especially positive BRCA2 gene mutations will most likely have a shorter effective run with the androgen-blocking drugs Xtandi® and Zytiga®.

Another lab test analyzing serum is called a "droplet digital PCR assay," and it can also help us determine which patients will best respond to those chemical agents, Xtandi® and Zytiga®. It should be noted that genetic markers are also important in light of the patient's family history. We want to know what the family history is with regard to other cancers. We can see that a patient's daughters may be prone to breast cancer or ovarian cancer; and now we are seeing colon and pancreatic cancers enter the picture in the spectrum related to prostate cancer. These cancers are essentially on the same page in our genetic makeup. Melanoma is also genetically related to prostate cancer, and all of these cancers may occur at increased frequency in the patient tested.

While genetic testing is important for the patient's siblings and children, (and also for the patient on occasion), there is even greater importance in sampling the actual cancerous tissue removed from the patient in order to identify somatic mutations. This is known as comprehensive genomic profiling (CGP). This test can help identify exactly which particular treatment may benefit the patient. AR-7 mutations suggest resistance to Xtandi®/Zytiga® while HRR gene mutations predict response to Lynparza® (olaparib).

REFERENCES AND ABSTRACTS

References

1. N Engl J Med 2009;360:1320-8. Prostate, Lung, Colorectal, and Ovarian Cancer Screening Trial (PLCO): Andriole GL, Grubb, III RL, Buys SS, et al. Mortality results from a randomized prostate-cancer screening trial. N Engl J Med 2009;360:1310-9.

2. European Randomized Study of Screening for Prostate Cancer (ERSPC): Schröder FH, Hugosson J, Roobol MJ, et al. Screening and prostate-cancer mortality in a randomized European study. N Engl J Med 2009;360:1320-8.

European Trial Abstract #1
Lancet Oncol. 2010 Aug;11 (8):725-32. Epub 2010 Jul 2.

Mortality results from the Göteborg randomised population-based prostate cancer screening trial.

Authors: Hugosson J, Carlsson S, Aus G, Bergdahl S, Khatami A, Lodding P, Pihl CG, Stranne J, Holmberg E, Lilja H.

Source: Department of Urology, Institute of Clinical Sciences, Sahlgrenska Academy at University of Göteborg, Sweden.

Abstract

METHODS: In December, 1994, 20,000 men born between 1930 and 1944, randomly sampled from the population register, were randomised by computer in a 1:1 ratio to either a screening group invited for PSA testing every 2 years (n=10,000) or to a control group not invited (n=10,000). Men in the screening group were invited up to the upper age limit (median 69, range 67-71 years) and only men with raised PSA concentrations were offered additional tests such as digital rectal examination and prostate biopsies. The primary endpoint was prostate cancer specific mortality, analysed according to the intention-to-screen principle. The study is ongoing, with men who have not reached the upper age limit invited for PSA testing. This is the first planned report on cumulative prostate-cancer incidence and mortality calculated up to Dec 31, 2008.

FINDINGS: In each group, 48 men were excluded from the analysis because of death or emigration before the randomization date, or prevalent prostate cancer. In men randomised to screening, 7578 (76%) of 9952 attended at least once. During a median follow-up of 14 years, 1138 men in the screening group and 718 in the control group were diagnosed with prostate cancer, resulting in a cumulative prostate cancer incidence of 12.7% in the screening group and 8.2% in the control group (hazard ratio 1.64; 95% CI 1.50-1.80; p<0.0001). The absolute cumulative risk reduction of death from prostate cancer at 14 years was 0.40% (95% CI 0.17-0.64), from 0.90% in the control group to 0.50% in the screening group. The rate ratio for death from prostate cancer was 0.56 (95% CI 0.39-0.82; p=0.002) in the screening compared with the control group. The rate ratio of death from prostate cancer for attendees compared with the control group was 0.44 (95% CI 0.28-0.68; p=0.0002). Overall, 293 (95% CI 177-799) men needed to be invited for screening and 12 to be diagnosed to prevent one prostate cancer death.

INTERPRETATION: This study shows that prostate cancer mortality was reduced almost by half over 14 years. However, the risk of over-diagnosis is substantial and the number needed to treat is at least as high as in breast-cancer screening programmes. The benefit of prostate cancer screening compares favourably to other cancer screening programs.

European Trial Abstract #2

N Engl J Med. 2012 Mar 15;366(11):981-90.

Prostate cancer mortality at 11 years of follow-up.

Authors: Schröder FH, Hugosson J, Roobol MJ, Tammela TL, Ciatto S, Nelen V, Kwiatkowski M, Lujan M, Lilja H, Zappa M, Denis LJ, Recker F, Páez A, Määttänen L, Bangma CH, Aus G, Carlsson S, Villers A, Rebillard X, van der Kwast T, Kujala PM, Blijenberg BG, Stenman UH, Huber A, Taari K, Hakama M, Moss SM, de Koning HJ, Auvinen A; ERSPC Investigators.

Source: Department of Urology, Erasmus University Medical Center, Rotterdam, The Netherlands.

Abstract

METHODS: The study involved 182,160 men between the ages of 50 and 74 years at entry, with a predefined core age group of 162,388 men 55 to 69 years of age. The trial was conducted in eight European countries. Men who were randomly assigned to the screening group were offered PSA-based screening, whereas those in the control group were not offered such screening. The primary outcome was mortality from prostate cancer.

RESULTS: After a median follow-up of 11 years in the core age group, the relative reduction in the risk of death from prostate cancer in the screening group was 21% ...and 29% after adjustment for noncompliance. The absolute reduction in mortality in the screening group was 0.10 deaths per 1000 person-years ...To prevent one death from prostate cancer at 11 years of follow-up, 1055 men would need to be invited for screening and 37 cancers would need to be detected. There was no significant between-group difference in all-cause mortality.

CONCLUSIONS: Analyses after 2 additional years of follow-up consolidated our previous finding that PSA-based screening significantly reduced mortality from prostate cancer but did not affect all-cause mortality.

2017 Retrospective Screening Study Abstract #3

Cancer, 2017 Dec 6.

The efficacy of prostate-specific antigen screening: Impact of key components in the ERSPC and PLCO trials.

de Koning HJ[1], Gulati R[2], Moss SM[3], Hugosson J[4], Pinsky PF[5], Berg CD[6], Auvinen A[7], Andriole GL[8], Roobol MJ[9], Crawford ED[10], Nelen V[11], Kwiatkowski M[12], Zappa M[13], Luján M[14], Villers A[15], de Carvalho TM[1], Feuer EJ[16], Tsodikov A[17], Mariotto AB[16], Heijnsdijk EAM[1], Etzioni R[2].

Sources

Department of Public Health, Erasmus Medical Center, Rotterdam, the Netherlands; Division of Public Health Sciences, Fred Hutchinson Cancer Research Institute, Seattle, Washington; Wolfson Institute, Queen Mary University of London, London, United Kingdom; Department of Urology, Sahlgrenska University Hospital, Goteborg, Sweden; Division of Cancer Prevention, National Cancer Institute, Bethesda, Maryland; Department of Radiation Oncology and Molecular Radiation Sciences, Johns Hopkins Medicine, Baltimore, Maryland; School of Health Sciences, University of Tampere, Tampere, Finland; Division of Urologic Surgery, Department of Surgery,

Washington University School of Medicine, St. Louis, Missouri; Department of Urology, Erasmus Medical Center, Rotterdam, the Netherlands; Urologic Oncology, University of Colorado, Denver, Colorado; Provinciaal Instituut voor Hygiene, Antwerp, Belgium; Department of Urology, Aarau Canton Hospital, Aarau, Switzerland; Unit of Epidemiology, Institute for Cancer Prevention, Florence, Italy; Urology Service, Infanta Cristina University Hospital, Complutense University of Madrid, Parla, Madrid, Spain; Department of Urology, Regional University Hospital Center, Lille, France; Division of Cancer Control and Population Sciences, National Cancer Institute, Bethesda, Maryland; Department of Biostatistics, University of Michigan, Ann Arbor, Michigan.

Abstract

BACKGROUND: The European Randomized Study of Screening for Prostate Cancer (ERSPC) demonstrated that prostate-specific antigen (PSA) screening significantly reduced prostate cancer mortality (rate ratio, 0.79; 95% confidence interval, 0.69-0.91). The US Prostate, Lung, Colorectal, and Ovarian (PLCO) trial indicated no such reduction but had a wide 95% CI (rate ratio for prostate cancer mortality, 1.09; 95% CI, 0.87-1.36). Standard meta-analyses are unable to account for key differences between the trials that can impact the estimated effects of screening and the trials' point estimates.

METHODS: The authors calibrated 2 microsimulation models to individual-level incidence and mortality data from 238,936 men participating in the ERSPC and PLCO trials. A cure parameter for the underlying efficacy of screening was estimated by the models separately for each trial. The authors changed step-by-step major known differences in trial settings, including enrollment and attendance patterns, screening intervals, PSA thresholds, biopsy receipt, control arm contamination, and primary treatment, to reflect a more ideal protocol situation and differences between the trials.

RESULTS: Using the cure parameter estimated for the ERSPC, the models projected 19% to 21% and 6% to 8%, respectively, prostate cancer mortality reductions in the ERSPC and PLCO settings. Using this cure parameter, the models projected a reduction of 37% to 43% under annual screening with 100% attendance and biopsy compliance and no contamination. The cure parameter estimated for the PLCO trial was 0.

CONCLUSIONS: The observed cancer mortality reduction in screening trials appears to be highly sensitive to trial protocol and practice settings. Accounting for these differences, the efficacy of PSA screening in the PLCO setting is not necessarily inconsistent with ERSPC results. Cancer 2017. © 2017 American Cancer Society.

APPENDIX B

A SURVEY OF CURRENTLY AVAILABLE BLOOD TESTS AND THEIR USES

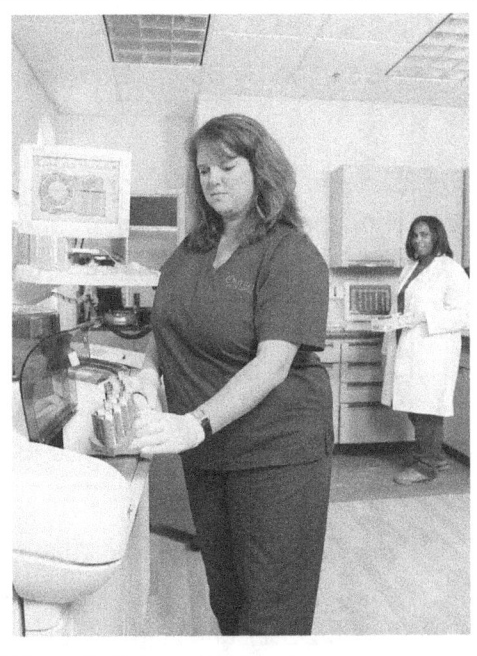

Depending on the specifics of the case, a number of tests may be indicated and are frequently utilized by the Dattoli team. Some of these tests, or markers, may be used to identify mutant tumor populations, or aggressive tumors in patients even without elevated PSAs. Markers of this type include NSE (Neuron Specific Enolase), CGA (Chromagranin A), and CEA (Carcinoembryonic Antigen). A number of other lab tests help to determine whether or not some form of hormonal therapy may be indicated either in the short term or at a later date. These tests include those that measure levels of Testosterone (total and bioavailable), DHT (dihydrotestosterone), DHEA-S (dehydroepiandrosterone sulphate), Estradiol, Prolactin, LH (Luteinizing Hormone) and Androstenedione.

Other procedures such as Urine Pyrilinks-D (Dpd), N-telopeptide (serum or urine), and Bone Specific Alkaline Phosphatase, are often used in addition to a Bone Mineral Density (BMD) test to establish a baseline for bone integrity. This is especially important for patients undergoing hormonal therapy, which can cause bone loss or resorption. We prefer a quantitative computerized tomography (QCT) scan over the Dual Energy X-ray Absorptiometry (DEXA) scan, as the QCT provides more accurate results. Additional tests such as a urine cytology study may be used to detect for other malignancies. Tests such as IGF-1 and 2L-6 may be included in a systemic evaluation.

Other Instruments and Associated Lab Tests

Immulite 2000 by Siemens Healthcare Diagnostics: PSA, 3rd generation PSA, PAP, Testosterone, SHGB, Estradiol, LH, Prolactin, Androstenedione, IGF-1, Vitamin B12, Folate

CellDyn 3200 by Abbott: CBC

Access 2 by Beckman/Coulter: BSAP and intact PTH

Envoy by Elitech: Electrolytes, Hepatic function, Kidney function, Glucose, LDH

Clinitek 500 by Bayer: Urinalysis

The following is a summary of blood tests that your doctor may order for pre-treatment diagnostic analysis and/or as part of your work-up before and during your course of treatment.

> **PSA (Prostatic Specific Antigen):** As discussed, the PSA assay is useful in detecting prostate cancer. As noted, the PSA may be temporarily elevated due to other factors such as sexual activity, prostatic massage, biopsy, infections, etc. The PSA test is also useful in detecting metastatic or persistent disease in patients following primary treatment for prostate cancer.
>
> **Testosterone, Total and Bioavailable Testosterone:** Testosterone and dihydrotestosterone (DHT) circulate in plasma either unbound, free (approximately 2-3%), or bound to plasma proteins. The binding proteins include the specific sex hormone-binding globulin (SHBG) and nonspecific proteins such as Albumin. The measurement of free testosterone or bioavailable testosterone more accurately reflects the level of bioactive testosterone than does the measurement of total serum testosterone. In aging men, total serum testosterone is often normal, while free testosterone or bioavailable testosterone is low. Testosterone levels are helpful in the assessment of androgen status in males. Increased testosterone levels are seen with androgen resistant prostate cancer. Decreased testosterone levels are seen with male hypogonadism, men with Cushing's disease, and men receiving glucocorticoid therapy.

SHBG (Sex Hormone Binding Globulin): SHBG is a beta-globulin that transports testosterone, dihydrotestosterone (DHT), and estradiol in plasma. It tightly binds approximately 60% of plasma testosterone and DHT. SHBG has the highest affinity for DHT and the lowest for Estradiol. The measurement of SHBG in serum can be useful in interpreting levels of testosterone.

Androstenedione: Produced by both the gonads and adrenals, androstenedione is an androgen having biologic activity less than that of testosterone (about one-third) but greater than DHEA. Levels are found to be higher in the morning.

PAP (Prostatic Acid Phosphatase): The prostate gland in men is a rich source of Acid Phosphatase. It normally contributes a small amount to the serum concentration. The clinical use of this prostate-specific fraction is in cases of prostate adenocarcinoma, where it is elevated most commonly in men with metastatic disease (about 60% of the cases). It is a much less sensitive test in men with localized disease (10-40% depending upon clinical grade). PAP will be transiently elevated following prostatic massage, needle biopsy, cystoscopy, and radiation.

DHEA-SO4: The DHEA-SO4 assay system measures the amount of dehydroepiandrosterone sulphate in human serum or plasma. This assay is an excellent direct indicator of adrenal androgen output, since DHEA-SO4 is almost exclusively synthesized by the adrenal cortex, and it is the most abundant steroid hormone in peripheral circulation.

Estradiol: Estradiol is a steroid estrogen compound secreted by the testes. Estradiol is elevated in cases of gynecomastia (breast enlargement and tenderness) which can be a side effect of hormonal therapy. Estradiol levels are decreased in cases of hypogonadism, a condition marked by a lowering of sex hormones and increased risk of osteoporosis (a decrease of bone mass and density).

Prolactin: This hormone stimulates the proliferation and growth of prostate cancer directly and by potentiating the action of testosterone. The hormonal therapy agent, Dostinex, blocks the production of Prolactin; therefore this level will be decreased while the patient is on this drug.

LH (Luteinizing Hormone): LH stimulates the Leydig cells of the testes to produce testosterone. If LH and follicle stimulating hormone (FSH) levels are elevated, primary gonadal failure may be indicated. LH will be decreased if the patient is on hormone therapy.

IGF-1 (Insulin-like Growth Factor-1 or Somatomedin C): IGF-1 is an important protein that is a signaling pathway in prostate cancer cells. It plays a major role in prostate cancer progression and development of hormone resistance.

BSAP (Bone Specific Alkaline Phosphatase): Although not totally understood, BSAP is believed to be involved in the mineralization of bone. The measurement of BSAP in serum provides information useful in the evaluation and treatment of patients with Paget's disease, osteoporosis, and prostate cancer metastases to bone.

DHT (Dihydrotestosterone): DHT is a primary androgenic hormone and is formed by the peripheral action of 5-alpha reductase on testosterone. The hormonal agents, Avodart® and Proscar®, inhibit 5-alpha reductase activity and reduce serum DHT concentrations.

NTX (N-Telopeptide, Cross-Linked): These biochemical markers of bone turnover exhibit significant changes during formation and resorption. These markers are useful in the management of patients' bone disease, allow earlier evaluation of treatment and are predictors of the risk of osteoporotic fractures.

NSE (Neuron Specific Enolase): NSE is a monoclonal antibody used as a tumor marker. Co-expression of NSE and Chromagranin–A are common in neuroendocrine neoplasms anywhere in the body, including the prostate and can indicate a mutated form of cancer.

CgA (Chromagranin A): CgA is an excellent supplemental marker in the diagnosis and management of patients with neuroendocrine tumors. Studies have shown elevated serum CgA levels in advanced stages of prostate cancer in patients receiving no hormonal treatment, yet an early rise in patients receiving such treatment. The assay provides a means of determining serum CgA levels for aiding in the diagnosis and prognosis of such neuroendocrine diseases, and for the monitoring of patients' response to therapy.

CK-ISO (Creatine Kinase Isoenzymes): Isoenzymes can be used to evaluate disorders other than cardiac or skeletal muscle. CK-BB activity can be evaluated in a variety of tumors (GI tract, prostate, testes, bladder, kidney, breast, ovary, uterus, CNS, leukemia, lymphomas, sarcomas).

IL-6 (Interleukin-6): IL-6 is a cytokine that regulates growth and differentiation of various types of malignant tumors, including prostate carcinomas. The level of IL-6 is elevated in sera of patients with metastatic prostate cancer.

Vitamin D 1,25 (Calcitriol): This test is used to determine if bone weakness, bone malformation, or abnormal metabolism of calcium (reflected by abnormal calcium, phosphorus or PTH tests) is occurring as a result of a deficiency or excess of vitamin D.

Calcitonin: This is a hormone known to participate in calcium and phosphorus metabolism. In particular, Calcitonin has the ability to decrease blood calcium levels by suppressing resorption of bone. It also inhibits reabsorption of calcium and phosphorus in the kidney, causing more to be lost in urine.

TSH (Thyroid Stimulating Hormone): TSH is used to diagnose a thyroid disorder in a person with symptoms.

PTH (Parathormone): PTH is measured to determine if PTH levels are responding normally to fluctuations in blood calcium levels, to distinguish the cause of calcium imbalances, and to evaluate parathyroid function.

CEA (Carcinoembryonic Antigen): CEA is used as a tumor marker and to monitor treatment of cancer patients.

CBC (Complete Blood Count): A CBC provides important information about the kinds and numbers of cells in the blood: red blood cells, white blood cells, and platelets.

- *WBC (White blood cell count):* A WBC is a count of the actual number of white blood cells per volume of blood. Both increases and decreases can be significant.

- *White blood cell differential:* This is used to look at the types of white blood cells present. There are five types of white cells: neutrophils, lymphocytes, monocytes, eosinophils and basophils. Each type has its own function in protecting us from infection.

- *RBC (Red blood cell count):* A count of the actual number of red cells per volume of blood. Both increases and decreases can point to abnormal conditions.

- **Hemoglobin:** Measures the amount of oxygen-carrying protein in the blood.

- **Hematocrit:** Measures the amount of space red blood cells take up in the blood.

- **Platelet count:** The number of platelets in a given volume of blood. Both increases and decreases can point to abnormal conditions of excess bleeding or clotting.

Comprehensive Metabolic Profile (CMP): The CMP is a group of 14 tests that gives your doctor important information about the current status of your kidneys, liver, and electrolyte and acid/base balance as well as of your blood sugar and blood proteins.

- **Glucose:** To determine if your blood glucose level is within normal range; to screen for, diagnose, and monitor diabetes, pre-diabetes and hypoglycemia.

- **Calcium:** Calcium is tested to screen for, diagnose and monitor a range of conditions relating to the bone, heart, nerves, kidney, and teeth.

- **Albumin:** To screen for liver disorders or kidney disease or to evaluate nutritional status.

- **Total Protein:** To determine your nutritional status or to screen for certain liver and kidney disorders as well as other diseases.

- **Sodium:** Used to monitor high or low blood pressure, dehydration, or edema.

- **Potassium:** This test is performed to diagnose levels of potassium that are too high (hyperkalemia) or too low (hypoklalemia). Potassium is important to heart function; it is a part of all complete routine evaluations.

- **CO_2:** CO_2 is part of an electrolyte panel to screen for an electrolyte or acid-base imbalance.

- **Chloride:** To determine if there is a problem with your body's acid-base and to monitor treatment.

- **BUN (Blood Urea Nitrogen):** The BUN level, usually along with Creatinine, is measured to evaluate kidney function as part of a routine panel or when someone has non-specific complaints, or when someone is prescribed certain medications.

- **Creatinine:** Creatinine is one of the waste products secreted by the kidneys. The test is used to determine if your kidneys are working normally. It is also used to monitor your kidney function while on certain drugs.

- **ALT, AST, ALP and Total Bilirubin:** These make up the rest of the 14 tests in this panel. They are defined below.

Hepatic Profile: This profile consists of the seven tests listed below. These tests are ordered for patients with symptoms or to monitor liver function during certain drug treatments.

- **ALT (Alanine aminotransferase):** An enzyme mainly found in the liver; the best test for detecting hepatitis.

- **AST (Aspartate aminotransferase):** An enzyme found in the liver, heart and other muscles.

- **ALP (Alkaline Phosphatase):** An enzyme related to the bile ducts; often increased when they are blocked.

- **Total Bilirubin:** Measures all the Bilirubin in the blood.

- **Direct Bilirubin:** Measures the form of Bilirubin made in the liver.

- **Albumin:** Measures the main protein made by the liver.

- **Total Protein:** Measures albumin and all other proteins in blood, including antibodies made to help fight infections.

- **Vitamin B12:** It is normally involved in the metabolism of every cell in the human body and energy production.

- **Folate:** This is a kind of Vitamin B found naturally in some foods like green vegetables and beans. Adequate levels of Folate have been linked to decreased risk of prostate cancer.

UA—Urinalysis: UA may consist of three testing phases.

1. Evaluating for color and clarity of the urine and testing the sample for: specific gravity (concentration of urine); pH (acidity of urine); protein (mainly albumin); glucose (sugar); ketones (products for fat metabolism); blood (hemoglobin); leukociyte esterase (suggests white blood cells in urine); nitrite (suggests bacteria present); bilirubin (possible liver disease); urobilinogen (possible liver disease).

2. A microscopic evaluation of the urine will be performed if indicated by any of the above results.

3. A culture and sensitivity analysis will be performed if indicated by microscopic evaluation.

Vitamin D 25: This is the stored form of Vitamin D. Decreased levels are linked to many disease states.

Vitamin D 1, 25: This is the physiologically active metabolite of Vitamin D. It has only limited use as an indicator of Vitamin D levels because its levels are influenced by other compounds such as calcium and PTH.

APPENDIX C

DECIDING WHAT IS BEST FOR YOU

Consult with your physician, and by all means, obtain second and third opinions whenever possible, preferably from physicians with different specialties. If you have already been to a urologist, it is worthwhile to visit a radiation oncologist or medical oncologist (those with experience with hormones and chemotherapy).

Join a support group such as Us TOO, or PAACT. If you belong to any of the computer on-line services, check out the medical and health bulletin boards and mailing lists for the latest information and announcements for prostate cancer patients. Keep your personal plan of action updated.

What to Remember

- Obtain all of the advice and counsel that you can, but keep in mind that the decisions are ultimately yours to make.

- Be positive—if you have been properly staged and treated, the odds are in your favor on not having a recurrence.

- If you should have a rising PSA over time after initial treatment, don't panic. Get further tests, and if appropriate, get a biopsy, preferably guided by color flow Doppler ultrasound.

- The secret to success with prostate cancer is catching the disease early, and that is also true for recurrence.

- If testing confirms cancer, learn all you can about your options. Get second and third opinions. Become informed and empowered. Become involved with solving your problem. It's your life and body. Go for it!

- Life is full of problems and challenges. Solve this problem like any other big problem:
    1. Identify the problem.
    2. Get all the facts to confirm that you have a problem.
    3. Learn what options are available to you and weigh them carefully.
    4. Choose a qualified doctor who is experienced and with whom you are comfortable.
    5. Initiate and follow through with the solution.
- Don't be afraid to ask for help from your spouse or partner, from your family and your friends. It is more important than ever for you to turn to loved ones to get the emotional and spiritual support you need. This disease can be a difficult struggle for us, but we are not alone, and our mental attitude, prayers and our fighting spirit really can make all the difference.

To be a cancer survivor, you must first be a cancer fighter!

APPENDIX D

GLOSSARY OF MEDICAL TERMS

3D-CRT (3-Dimensional Conformal Radiation Therapy): See Conformal Radiotherapy.

5-alpha reductase (5-AR): an enzyme that converts testosterone to dihydrotestosterone (DHT).

Adenocarcinoma: A cancer originating in glandular tissue. Prostate cancer is classified as adenocarcinoma of the prostate.

Adjuvant: An additional treatment used to increase the effectiveness of the primary therapy. Radiation therapy and hormonal therapy are often used as adjuvant treatments following a radical prostatectomy. Compare Neoadjuvant.

Agonist: A chemical substance that combines with a receptor on a cell and initiates an activity or reaction. See LHRH analogs.

Algorithm: A step-by-step procedure for solving a problem or accomplishing some end, especially by a computer.

Analog: A man-made chemical compound that is structurally similar to one produced naturally by the body. See LHRH analogs.

Anastomotic stricture: narrowing, usually by scarring, of an anastomotic suture line.

Androgen: A hormone that produces male characteristics. See testosterone.

Androgen ablation therapy: A therapy designed to inhibit the body's production of testosterones.

Androgen-dependent cells: Prostate cancer cells which are nourished by male hormones and therefore are capable of being destroyed by hormone deprivation (also known as androgen-sensitive cells).

Androgen-independent cells: Prostate cancer cells which are not dependent on male hormones and therefore do not respond to hormonal therapy (also known as androgen-insensitive cells).

Anesthetic: A drug that produces general or local loss of physical sensations, particularly pain. A "spinal" is the injection of a local anesthetic into the area surrounding the spinal cord.

Aneuploid: Having an abnormal number of chromosomes, as revealed by ploidy analysis. Aneuploid prostate cancer cells tend not to respond well to androgen deprivation therapy (ADT).

Angiogenesis: The body's formation of new blood vessels. Some anti-cancer drugs work by blocking angiogenesis, thus preventing blood from reaching and nourishing a tumor.

Antagonist: A chemical substance in the body that acts to reduce the physiological activity of another chemical substance.

Antiandrogens: Drugs such as Casodex that block the activity of androgens produced by the adrenal glands at the cellular receptor sites. Androgens can block or neutralize the effects of testosterone and DHT on prostate cancer cells.

Antibody: A protein produced by the body that counteracts the toxic effects of a foreign substance, organism, or disease within the body.

Antigen: A foreign substance such as a virus or bacterium that causes an immune response or the formation of an antibody.

Antineoplastic: Inhibits growth and proliferation of cancer cells.

Antioxidants: Any substances which delay the process of oxidation in the body.

Apoptosis: The normal molecular mechanism which governs the life span of cells so that they die in a very organized way. Cancerous cells are resistant to normal apoptosis.

Benign: A non-cancerous condition. *See also Benign Prostatic Hypertrophy.*

Benign Prostatic Hypertrophy (BPH): Also called Benign Prostatic Hyperplasia, BPH is a non-cancerous condition of the prostate that results in a growth of tumorous tissue and increase in the size of the prostate.

Biopsy: A procedure involving the removal of tissue from the body of the patient. Removed tissue is typically examined microscopically by a pathologist in order to make a precise diagnosis of the patient's condition.

Bone scan: An imaging technique used to detect bone metastases, which appear as "hot spots" on the film. It is far more sensitive than the conventional x-ray.

BPH: *See Benign Prostatic Hypertrophy.*

Brachytherapy: A form of radiation therapy in which radioactive seeds are implanted into the prostate to deliver radiation directly to the tumor. Also referred to as seed implantation, or seeding.

Cancer: A cellular malignancy typically forming tumors. Unlike benign tumors, these tend to invade surrounding tissues and spread to distant sites of the body.

Carcinoma: A malignant tumor made up chiefly of epithelial cells, or those cells that form the lining of an organ or cavity. See *Adenocarcinoma*.

Castrate Range: The level of the body's testosterone after orchiectomy (also referred to as castration). This is the range or level, which is used by physicians as a point of comparison for those drugs, which attempt to decrease the testosterone level.

CAT Scan (or CT Scan): *See Computer Tomography.*

cGy: Abbreviation for centigray; a unit of radiation equivalent to the older unit called a "rad."

Chemotherapy: The treatment of cancer using chemicals that deter the growth of cancer cells.

Collimator: A device that organizes radiation such that only parallel rays or beams emanate.

Combination Hormonal Therapy (CHT): Also referred to as Combined Hormonal Blockade (CHB), or Combined Androgen Deprivation Therapy (ADT). The preferred term is ADT, often designated with a number referring to the number of agents used (i.e., monotherapy ADT, ADT2, ADT3). This combined therapy can utilize a number of mechanisms, including surgical or medical ADT, antiandrogens, 5-alpha reductase inhibitors, estrogenic compounds, agents that block adrenal androgen production, and agents that decrease the receptivity of the androgen receptor.

Combination Therapy: Refers generally to any combination of treatment modalities used to treat prostate cancer.

Computer Tomography: Computer generated cross-sectional images of a portion of the body. Also called CT or CAT scan.

Conformal Radiotherapy: A radiation treatment conforming precisely to the size and shape of the prostate, with the use of computerized planning and state-of-the-art imaging techniques. 3-Dimensional Conformal Radiation Therapy (3D-CRT) utilizes this sophisticated approach to treatment planning, as does the even more advanced Intensity Modulated Radiation Therapy (IMRT).

Cryosurgery (also referred to as Cryotherapy or Cryoablation): The freezing of tissue with the use of liquid nitrogen or Argon gas probes. When used to treat prostate cancer, the cryoprobes are guided by transrectal ultrasound.

Cytokine: Any of a class of immunoregulatory substances that are secreted by cells of the immune system.

DHT (dihydrotestosterone): The active form of the male hormone, testosterone, produced after testosterone is transformed by an enzyme known as 5-alpha reductase.

Diagnosis: Evaluation of a patient's symptoms and/or test results, with the intent of identifying and verifying the existence of any underlying disease or abnormal condition.

Digital Rectal Examination (DRE): A procedure in which the physician inserts a gloved, lubricated finger into the rectum to examine the prostate gland for signs of cancer.

DNA (Deoxyribonucleic Acid): A complex protein that is the carrier of genetic information that determines the physical development and growth of living organisms.

Doppler Ultrasound Technique: A machine that sends out ultrasonic waves that pick up the velocity of blood flow through the veins and are transmitted as sound to make an image.

Doubling Time: The time it takes for a tumor or cancerous focus to double in size.

Downsizing: The use of hormonal therapy or other forms of intervention to reduce tumor volume prior to primary, curative treatment.

Downstaging: The use of hormonal therapy or other forms of intervention to lower the clinical stage of prostate cancer prior to primary, curative treatment.

Ejaculatory Ducts: The tubular passages through which semen reaches the prostatic urethra during orgasm.

Ejaculation: The release of semen through the penis during orgasm.

Endorectal MRI: Magnetic resonance imaging of the prostate gland using a probe inserted into the rectum. Dynamic Contrast Enhanced MRI is the most effective form of magnetic resonance imaging.

Enzyme: A chemical substance produced by living cells that causes chemical reactions to take place while not being changed itself.

Erectile Dysfunction (also referred to as ED or impotence): The loss of ability to produce and/or sustain an erection sufficient for intercourse.

Estrogen: A female sex hormone that can be used as a form of therapy to inhibit the production of testosterone in patients diagnosed with prostate cancer.

External Beam Radiation Therapy (EBRT): A form of radiation therapy that utilizes radiation delivered by an external source (machine) and directed at a target area to be radiated. In contrast to EBRT, brachytherapy utilizes radiation sources (seeds) that are internal, implanted in the target tissue. EBRT may use conventional photons, protons, neutrons or electrons.

Extraprostatic Extension: Used to describe prostate cancer that has spread outside the prostate gland.

False Negative: An erroneous negative test result. For example, an imaging test that fails to show the presence of a cancer tumor later found by biopsy to be present in the patient is said to have returned a false negative result.

False Positive: A positive test result that mistakenly identifies a state or condition that does not in fact exist.

Feraheme (Ferumoxytol): A ferromagnetic nanoparticle which is taken up by normal macrophages with the lymph nodes.

Fistula: With regard to prostate cancer, an abnormal passage due to injury or disease that connects an abscess or hollow organ to the surface of the body or to another hollow organ. If there is significant damage to the rectal wall proximate to the bladder, a fistula may occur between the bladder and rectum.

Flare Reaction: A testosterone surge caused by the initial use of an LHRH analog, causing a temporary increase of tumor growth and symptoms (known as clinical flare), or an increase in PSA (biochemical flare).

Foley Catheter: A catheter inserted in the penis and threaded through the urethra to the bladder where it is held in place with a tiny, inflated balloon. It removes urine from the bladder and can be used to irrigate the urethra and prevent blood clots.

Free PSA: PSA that is unattached to any major protein in the blood. Free PSA is associated with benign prostate growth. The percentage of free PSA is derived by dividing the free-PSA level by the total-PSA x 100. Studies have show that men with free PSA % > 25% were at low risk for prostate cancer, while men with PSA % < 10% were at high risk for having prostate cancer.

Frozen Section: A technique in which removed tissue is frozen, cut into thin slices, and stained for microscopic examination. A pathologist can rapidly complete a frozen section analysis, and for this reason, it is commonly used during surgery to quickly provide the surgeon with vital information.

Gland: An aggregation of cells (a structure or organ) that secretes a substance for use or discharge from the body.

Gland Volume: The size in cubic centimeters (cc) or grams of the prostate gland.

Gleason Score: A widely used method for classifying the cellular differentiation of cancerous tissue. The less the cancerous cells appear like normal cells, the more malignant the cancer. Two grades of 1-5, identifying the two most common degrees of differentiation present in the examined tissue sample, are added together to produce the Gleason score. High numbers indicate greater differentiation and more aggressive cancer. The grading system is named after its originator, Donald Gleason, M.D.

Globulin: Any of a number of simple proteins that occur widely in plant and animal tissues.

Gynecomastia: A side effect involving breast enlargement and tenderness, associated with various hormonal therapies that increase the level of estrogens in the body.

HDR brachytherapy: High Dose Rate brachytherapy involves the temporary insertion of radioactive iridium isotopes into the prostate gland using transrectal ultrasound guidance.

Hematuria: Blood in the urine.

Hereditary: Inherited genetically from parents and earlier generations.

Holistic Medicine: Medical care, which considers the patient as a whole, including his or her physical, mental, emotional, spiritual, social and economic needs.

Hormone: A substance produced by one tissue or gland and transported by the bloodstream to another to effect or regulate physiological activity such as metabolism and growth.

Hormonal therapy: Cancer treatment involving the blockage of hormone production by surgical or chemical means. Because prostate cancer is usually dependent on male hormones to grow, hormonal therapy can be an effective means of alleviating symptoms and retarding the development of the disease.

Hormone refractory prostate cancer: Prostate cancer that is androgen independent, and therefore, unresponsive to hormonal therapies.

Hot Flash: A side effect of some forms of hormonal therapy, experienced as a sudden rush of warmth to the face, neck, and upper body.

Imaging: Radiology techniques that are often computer-enhanced and allow the physician to visualize areas inside the body that would not normally be visible.

Impotence: *See Erectile Dysfunction.*

Incontinence: A loss of urinary control. There are various kinds and degrees of incontinence. Overflow incontinence is a condition in which the bladder retains urine after voiding. As a consequence, the bladder remains full most of the time, resulting in involuntary seepage of urine from the bladder. Stress incontinence is the involuntary discharge of urine when there is increased pressure upon the bladder, as in coughing or straining to lift heavy objects. Total incontinence is the failure of ability to voluntarily exercise control over the sphincters of the bladder neck and urethra, resulting in total loss of retentive ability.

Inflammation: Redness or swelling caused by injury or infection.

Informed Consent: Permission to proceed given by a patient after being fully informed of the purposes and potential consequences of a medical procedure.

Intensity Modulated Radiation Therapy (IMRT): The most recent state-of-the-art, computer-aided technique for delivering higher doses of radiation more accurately than either conventional External Beam Radiation or Conformal Radiation. The most advanced form of IMRT is Dynamic Adaptive Radiotherapy (DART).

Intermittent Androgen Deprivation (IAD): A temporary discontinuation of hormonal therapy that allows for a return to natural testosterone production in order to spare the patient from symptoms associated with androgen deprivation. Also referred to as Intermittent Hormonal Therapy (IHT).

Intravenous Pyelogram (IVP): A test that utilizes the injection of a special dye to check for injury or the spread of cancer to the kidneys and bladder.

Investigational: A drug or procedure allowed by the FDA for use in clinical trails, but not necessarily reimbursed.

Isodose Line: A line or two-dimensional shape that circumscribes an area receiving a radiation dose greater than or equal to a specified amount.

Laparoscopic Lymphadenectomy: The removal of pelvic lymph nodes with a laparoscope via four small incisions in the lower abdomen.

LH (Luteinizing Hormone): A chemical signal originating in the pituitary gland that causes the testes to make testosterone.

LHRH Analogs (or LHRH Agonists): Synthetic compounds that are chemically similar to Luteinizing Hormone Releasing Hormone (LHRH), used to suppress testicular production of testosterone. The most commonly prescribed LHRH analogs are Lupron® and Zoldex® Eligard® and Trelstar®. *See also Luteinizing Hormone-Releasing Hormone (LHRH).*

LHRH Antagonist: A chemical agent that blocks the LHRH receptor without the testosterone surge associated with LHRH analogs. LHRH antagonists include Abarelix (Plenaxis®).

Linear Accelerator: A high energy x-ray machine generating radiation fields for external beam radiation therapy. These machines are typically mounted with a collimator (or multileaf collimator) in a gantry that rotates vertically around the patient being treated.

Localized Prostate Cancer: Cancer that is confined to the prostate gland, and therefore, considered curable.

Luteinizing Hormone-Releasing Hormone (LHRH): A chemical signal originating in the hypothalamus that causes the pituitary to make LH, which in turn stimulates the testicles to make testosterone.

Lymphadenectomy: The removal and examination of lymph nodes to precisely diagnose and stage cancer. *See also Laparascopic Lymphadenectomy.*

Lymph Node: A small, bean-shaped mass of tissue located throughout the body along the vessels of the lymphatic system. The lymph nodes filter out bacteria and other toxins, as well as cancer cells.

Magnetic Resonance Imaging (MRI): A painless, non-invasive technique using strong magnetic fields to produce detailed images of internal body structures. An MRI scan usually takes about 45 minutes per site.

Malignancy: A tumorous growth of cancer cells.

Malignant: Having the invasive and metastatic properties of cancer. Tending to become progressively worse and to result in death.

Margin: *See Surgical Margin.*

Metalloprotease Inhibitors: Drugs used to suppress the body's production of certain enzymes.

Metastasis: The spread of cancer, by way of the blood stream or lymphatic system, beyond the boundaries of the organ or structure where the cancer originated. Metastases is the plural. Metastatic refers to the characteristics associated with cancer that has spread or a secondary tumor.

Metastatic Work-Up: A group of tests, including bone scans, x-rays, and blood tests, to ascertain whether cancer has metastasized.

Monoclonal Antibody (mAb): An antibody that is directed against one specific protein (antigen).

Morbidity: Unhealthy consequences and complications resulting from treatment.

MRI: *See Magnetic Resonance Imaging.*

Nadir: The lowest point. Doctors sometimes use this as a verb to describe return of cancer or treatment failure. The PSA nadir refers to a minimum PSA value that should be maintained after treatment if the cancer has been successfully eradicated.

Necrosis: Death of cells or tissues caused by disease or injury.

Neoadjuvant: The use of a different type of therapy before primary, curative treatment. For example, neoadjuvant Androgen Deprivation Therapy is often used prior to radiation therapy or radical surgery, with the intent of improving the effectiveness of the primary treatment by reducing the size of the tumor and/or prostate gland.

Nerve-sparing: A procedure used during radical prostatectomy in which the surgeon attempts to save the nerves (neurovascular bundles) that allow for normal sexual functions.

Neurovascular Bundles: Strands of interwoven nerves and veins that run down the side of the prostate. The bundles contain microscopic nerves that are essential for erection; they also contain arteries and veins. Cutting the nerves in the bundles during surgery, or otherwise harming them in another procedure, usually renders the patient impotent.

Nocturia: Getting up at night to urinate.

Non-invasive: Not involving any incision in the body.

Oncogenes: Genes associated with tumor growth.

Oncology: The branch of medical science dealing with tumors. A medical oncologist is a specialist in the study of cancerous tumors.

Organ-confined Disease (OCD): Prostate cancer that is confined to the prostate gland, as indicated clinically or pathologically.

Orchiectomy: A simple operation that involves surgical removal of the testicles, which produce most of the body's testosterone.

Osteoporosis: A decrease in bone mass and density causing fragility and porosity.

Overstaging: An assessment of an overly high clinical stage at initial diagnosis.

Palliative: Affording symptomatic pain relieve but not cure or remission.

Palpable: Capable of being felt when examined by touch or manipulation.

PAP: *See Prostatic Acid Phosphatase.*

Pathologist: A doctor who specializes in the examination of cells and tissues removed from the body.

PBRT:
See Proton Beam Radiation Therapy.

Perineum: The area of the body between the anus and scrotum. A perineal procedure uses this area as the point of entry into the body.

Perineural Invasion: Describing cancer, which has spread from the prostate to the nerve bundles.

Periprostatic: Relating to the soft tissues immediately proximate to the prostate gland.

Photon: The quantum of electromagnetic energy, described as having zero mass and no electric charge. X-rays are high energy photons.

Placebo: A sugar pill often taken by participants in a medical study. Patients taking a placebo are compared to patients taking actual medications.

Ploidy Analysis: A pathological analysis to determine the number of sets of chromosomes in a cell.

Proctitis: Inflammation of the rectum.

Prognosis: A forecast of the course of a disease and future prospects of the patient.

Progression: A change in the status of the cancer indicating the condition has progressed and worsened.

Pro-oxidant: A term to describe substances that aid in oxidation.

ProstaScint® Scan: An imaging technique sometimes used determine whether or not cancer has spread to distant sites by using monoclonal antibodies.

Prostate Capsule: It was once thought that the prostate gland was surrounded by a clearly identifiable capsule, but pathological studies have shown there is no capsule as such. The gland exists within a fat plane.

Prostatectomy: The surgical removal of part or all of the prostate gland.

Prostate Specific Antigen (PSA): A blood test that measures a substance manufactured solely by prostate gland cells. An elevated reading indicates an abnormal condition of the prostate gland, either benign or malignant. It is presently the most sensitive tumor marker for the identification and monitoring of prostate cancer.

Prostatic Acid Phosphatase (PAP): An enzyme produced by the prostate that is elevated (3.0 or higher) in many patients when prostate cancer has spread beyond the prostate.

Prostatitis: An infection or inflammation of the prostate gland that is treatable with medications.

Proton Beam Radiation Therapy (PBRT): A form of radiation therapy that utilizes protons as the source of energy (as opposed to X-rays or neutrons).

PSA: *See Prostate Specific Antigen.*

PSA Bounce (or PSA Bump): A rise in PSA level after first having a reduction in PSA after radiation therapy.

PSA Nadir: The lowest PSA value after a particular treatment.

PSA Velocity (PSAV): The rate of increase of the PSA level, expressed as nanograms per milliliter per year.

Radiation Therapy (RT): The use of high energy rays to kill cancer cells and malignant tissue.

Radiation Urethritis: Inflammation of the urethra caused by radiation therapy.

Radical Prostatectomy: An operation to remove the entire prostate gland and seminal vesicles.

Radiosensitivity: The degree to which a type of cancer responds to radiation therapy.

RBA or Relative Biological Effectiveness: A scale used to compare the intensity of radiation associated with various atomic particles.

Receptor: A cellular docking site that interacts with a specific protein or enzyme (called a ligand). The interaction typically leads to the synthesis of other substances such as proteins, hormones or enzymes.

Recurrence: Return of the cancer following remission or treatment intended as curative. Local recurrence indicates a return of the cancer at the site of origin. Distant recurrence indicates the appearance of one or more metastases of the disease.

Refractory: A term indicating that the cancer no longer responds to the current therapy.

Remission: Complete or partial disappearance of the signs and symptoms of the disease. The period during which a disease remains under control, without progressing. Even complete remission does not necessarily indicate cure.

Resection: The surgical removal of a part of an organ or structure.

Risk: The probability that a particular event will or will not happen.

RP: *See Radical Prostatectomy.*

RT: *See Radiation Therapy.*

Rx: The standard abbreviation for prescription.

Salvage Treatment: A medical term for "Plan B." It means a patient must undergo another form of treatment because the first therapy was not successful. Salvage therapy may incur a higher rate of side effects.

Saw Palmetto: A nutrient extracted from the saw palmetto shrub, which is considered by some to aid the body's immune system.

Seed Implantation (SI): A minimally invasive procedure by which radioactive seeds are implanted into the prostate gland to destroy cancer. Also referred to as seeding and brachytherapy.

Selenium: A non-metallic element thought to be beneficial as a nutrient; it is often included in multivitamin supplements.

Seminal Vesicles: Glands that, like the prostate, support male reproduction. Fluid secreted by these glands regulates the consistency of semen.

Side Effect: A reaction to a treatment or medication, usually referring to an undesirable effect.

Sphincter: A circular muscle which contracts to close an orifice. The urethral sphincter squeezes the urethra shut, providing urinary control.

Staging: The testing process by which the extent and severity of a known cancer is evaluated according to an established system of classification. It is used to help determine appropriate therapy. See *TNM Staging and Whitmore-Jewett Staging*.

Surgical Margin: The outer edge of the tissue removed during a radical prostatectomy. The surgical margin may be "negative," indicating that no cancer is present and a better prognosis, or "positive," indicating that not all of the cancer has been removed.

Systemic: Throughout the body and affecting the entire body.

T-Cell: An immune system cell or lymphocyte that directs an immune response to malignant or infected cells.

Testes: Two male reproductive glands located inside the scrotum. The testes are the primary sources for testosterone. Also called testicles.

Testosterone: A male sex hormone chiefly produced by the testicles.

Thrombotic: Causing or relating to blood clotting.

TNM Staging: The most widely used classification system for evaluating the extent of prostate cancer. TNM refers to tumor, nodes and metastases. See *Staging*.

Transrectal: Through the rectum.

Transurethral: Through the urethra.

Transrectal Ultrasonography: See *Ultrasound*.

Transurethral Resection of the Prostate (TURP): A surgical procedure to remove tissue obstructing the urethra. The technique involves the insertion of an instrument called a resectoscope into the penile urethra, and is intended to relieve obstruction of urine flow due to enlargement of the prostate.

Tumor: An excessive growth of cells that is caused by uncontrolled and disorderly cell replacement. Abnormal tissue growth may be benign or malignant. See also *Benign, Malignant*.

TURP: See *Transurethral Resection of the Prostate*.

Ultrasound (Transrectal Ultrasonography): A painless, non-invasive diagnostic imaging technique using sound waves to create an echo pattern that reveals the structure of organs and tissues. It does not use x-rays.

Understaging: An overly low assessment of clinical stage at diagnosis.

Urethra: The tube that carries urine from the bladder and semen from the prostate out of the body through the penis.

Urologist: A physician who specializes in the diagnosis and the medical and surgical treatment of problems in the urinary and male reproductive systems.

USPIO: This technology uses ultrasmall superparamagnetic iron oxide (USPIO) as an MRI contrast agent for the identification of cancer metastasis in lymph nodes.

Vasectomy: A surgical procedure to render a man sterile by cutting the vas deferens, thus eliminating the passage of sperm from the testes to the prostate.

Vasoactive: Causing the dilation or constriction of blood vessels.

Vesicle: A small sac containing fluid, as in seminal vesicles.

Whitmore-Jewett Staging: A classification system for evaluating the extent of prostate cancer. This system is less widely used for the designation of stage than is TNM staging.

X-rays: High energy radiation that can be used at low levels of intensity to make images of the body's internal structures, or at high intensity for radiation therapy.

APPENDIX E

THE WARNING SIGNS OF PROSTATE CANCER

There are often no warning signs of prostate cancer. In some cases the following symptoms may indicate the presence of the disease. However, please be aware that these symptoms may also be due to benign conditions of the prostate, or other conditions entirely unrelated to prostate cancer:

- Elevated or rising PSA
- Abnormal Digital Rectal Exam
- Blood in urine
- Pain or difficulty urinating
- Increased urge to urinate, especially at night
- Hesitant or intermittent urinary flow
- Pain or discomfort in area of prostate
- Unusual and unexplained weight loss
- Continual pain in lower back, hips or pelvis
- Increased voiding urgency
- Inability to urinate
- Trouble having or keeping an erection (erectile dysfunction)
- Weakness or numbness in the legs or feet

ABOUT THE AUTHOR

Michael J. Dattoli, MD

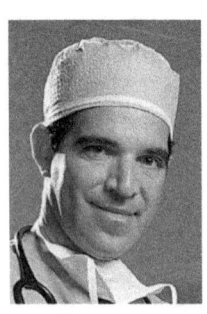

Michael J. Dattoli, MD, is a board-certified radiation oncologist with well over two decades of brachytherapy experience and has performed thousands of prostate implant procedures. He is considered the foremost pioneer in the field, optimizing brachytherapy designs to maximize tumor eradication and minimize symptoms. He has also been the leading trailblazer in the development of Dynamic Adaptive Radiotherapy (DART), utilizing all of the state-of-the-art modalities associated with 4-Dimensional Image-Guided Intensity Modulated Radiotherapy (3D-IMRT). Dr. Dattoli has successfully applied the same technologies to other forms of cancer, including breast, head and neck, GI, GYN, sarcomas and lung malignancies. He is a noted author and speaker in this complex field of medicine.

Dr. Dattoli attended the University of California at Berkeley and was the Valedictorian of his class at Vassar College; he earned his medical degree at Mount Sinai School of Medicine, Radiation Oncology at New York University Medical Center, then distinguished himself at Memorial Sloan-Kettering Cancer Center and New York Hospital-Cornell University Medical Center, as the Special Fellow in Brachytherapy. He was appointed Associate Professor in Brachytherapy and Radiation Oncology at Memorial Sloan-Kettering Cancer Center in New York and at New York Hospital-Cornell University Medical Center prior to relocating to Florida.

Dr. Dattoli also serves on multiple journal editorial review boards. Government appointments include "The Prostate Cancer Task Force" in Florida and consultant to the "Washington Oncology Roundtable Advisory Committee". He was selected by the International Association of Oncologists as a Leading Physician of the World and top Brachytherapist.

THE DATTOLI CANCER FOUNDATION MISSION

The Dattoli Cancer Foundation, sponsor of the Prostate Cancer Resource Network, is a 501(c)(3), tax-exempt charitable organization, whose mission is

- ◆ to raise awareness of the wide-spread incidence of Prostate Cancer and the need for early and annual screenings;

- ◆ to provide information and support to men newly diagnosed with Prostate Cancer as well as to those with recurrent Prostate Cancer, and

- ◆ to foster research into better diagnostic tools and treatment options for Prostate Cancer.

Gifts to the Dattoli Foundation make possible publications like this one, and are welcomed anytime. A copy of the official registration and financial information may be obtained from the Division of Consumer Services by calling toll-free (800-435-7352) within the state. Registration does not imply endorsement, approval or recommendations by the state.

Dattoli Cancer Foundation
2803 Fruitville Road
Sarasota, FL 34237
941/365-5599
800/915-1001
fax: 941/332-2317
www.dattolifoundation.org

ORDER MORE BOOKLETS IN THE SERIES

This *Prostate Cancer Essentials for Survival* booklet was published by the Dattoli Cancer Foundation. For a complete list of booklets in the series and ordering information, please visit the Dattoli Cancer Center Book Shelf at dattoli.com/book-shelf. Current titles include::

- ✓ Coping with Prostate Cancer Recurrence
- ✓ Conquering Prostate Cancer with DART and Brachytherapy
- ✓ The Dattoli Prostate Cancer Challenge: Evaluating All Your Treatment Options
- ✓ The Facts: Comparing Prostate Cancer Treatment Options
- ✓ Dynamic Adaptive Radiotherapy
- ✓ Image-Guided Prostate Biopsy: When, Why and What to Expect
- ✓ Dosimetry and Prostate Cancer Radiotherapy
- ✓ Advanced Imaging for Prostate Cancer: A Primer on 3D Color-Flow Power Doppler Ultrasound, Multiparametric MRI and CT Fusion Techniques
- ✓ Radiation Safety and Prostate Cancer: Need You Be Concerned?
- ✓ Hormonal Therapy for Prostate Cancer: The Benefits and Risks
- ✓ Lymph Node Positive Prostate Cancer: Advanced Diagnostics and Treatment
- ✓ The Dattoli Blue Ribbon Prostate Cancer Solution: How to Survive and Thrive Without Surgery

www.ingramcontent.com/pod-product-compliance
Lightning Source LLC
Chambersburg PA
CBHW070213230526
45471CB00002B/936